Moulds and Mycotoxins in Poultry Diseases

Prof. S.M. Mohiuddin (Retd.)
B.V. Sc., M.V. Sc. Ph.D. (Path.)
Department of Pathology,
College of Veterinary Science,
Andhra Pradesh Agricultural University,
Rajendranagar, Hyderabad - 500 030, India

International Book Distributing Co.
(Publishing Division)

Published by

INTERNATIONAL BOOK DISTRIBUTING CO.

(Publishing Division)
Khushnuma Complex Basement
7, Meerabai Marg (Behind Jawahar Bhawan)
Lucknow 226 001 U.P. (INDIA)
Tel. : 91-522-2209542, 2209543, 2209544, 2209545
Fax : 0522-4045308
E-Mail : ibdco@airtelbroadband.in

First Edition 2007

Price MAXIMUM RETAIL PRICE INCLUSIVE OF ALL TAXES ₹ 850.00

ISBN 81-8189-123-6

Composed & Designed at :

Panacea Computers
3rd Floor, Agarwal Sabha Bhawan
Subhash Mohal,
Sadar Lucknow-226 002
Tel : 0522-2483312, 93359 27082
E-mail : prasgupt@rediffmail.com, prasgupt@hotmail.com

Printed at:

Salasar Imaging Systems
C-7/5, Lawrence Road Industrial Area
Delhi - 110 035
Tel. : 011-27185653, 9810064311

PREFACE

During the last three decades poultry production has made a tremendous progress. The improved layer population have exceeded a million during 1961 to 67 million in 1986, which resulted in increased egg production from 360 million to 1425 million. Similarly the broiler production have achieved tremendous increase from 4 millions 1971 to 95 millions during 1986. This transition of poultry farming from a backyard rearing to a large-scale intensive poultry rearing with investment running into millions of rupees is due to embarking upon large scale import of germplasm and technical know how. However, during recent years the growth is not as high as it was for many unknown diseases have been faced by the poultry.

The recent years have shown that mycosis and mycotoxicosis have been assuming considerable importance in aetiology of many unknown diseases in poultry. The fungi are ubiquitous in nature and there are frequent opportunities available in our Indian agro-climatic conditions for their growth during harvest and storage to elaborate their toxin. The problem of mycotoxicosis in the health of human and livestock has assumed a much importance, only after the outbreak of Turkey X disease during 1960.

The heavy economic losses faced by the in poultry industry either by death of birds or by production losses is due to the feeding of mouldy feed. The mycotoxicosis is also responsible for bruising in broilers thus lowering the carcass value, immuno-suppressive effects. Increase in the requirement of certain nutrients leading to deficiency syndrome, and finally the toxic metabolites are excreted through meat and eggs leading to human health hazards.

The problem of moulds and mycotoxicosis in poultry is a worldwide phenomenon and to understand the magnitude of mycotoxicosis problem in poultry, its biochemical, mechanism of action effects on different organs and their prevention, the present summer institute/short course has been designed in the form of lectures from eminent persons in that area, practical demonstrations and field visits. The lectures have been designed to provide general information on mycotoxins, its effect on poultry, and its control. I hope that the information noted with all sincerity and purpose of education will increase awareness of the problem of moulds and mycotoxicosis in poultry.

Rajendranagar

S.M. MOHIUDDIN

Contents

CHAPTER

1 THE IMPACT OF AFLATOXINS OF POULTRY INDUSTRY

Dr. P.V. Rao,
Professor & Univ. Head, Department of Poultry Science, CVSc,
APAU, R'nagar, Hyderabad-500 030.

INTRODUCTION

Aflatoxins in poultry feeds have long been associated with impaired performance of poultry ranging from decrease in weight gains, drop in egg production and break in immunity. The economic losses in terms of broiler weights or egg output have been accurately estimated. However, because of the ubiquitous incidence of the condition, the losses could be considerable.

In India, our interest in the realm of animal production vis-a-vis aflatoxicosis is more recent. And naturally our understanding of the subject is far from complete.

Mode of action

Aflatoxins exert their effect in poultry (and other animals) is more than on way. Published reports say that aflatoxins, as also other mycotoxins, exert their effect more by interfering with normal metabolic pathways. The ones that are established among these include:

Inhibition of protein synthesis

Adverse effect on fat metabolism

Inhibition of enzyme systems involved in carbohydrate

metabolism and energy release

More grossly, the lesions include:

Liver tumors, kidney enlargement, haemorrhage in intestines, bursal regression etc, while many of these are non-specific, bursal regression is characteristic of avian aflatoxicosis.

Classification

There are many mycotoxins and some of which are more toxic than others. Aflatoxins as a group are more commonly encountered than others. Depending upon the pathological changes they bring about in the body changes, they are grouped as hepatotoxic, nephrotoxic etc. Aflatoxins are primarily hepatotoxins, the most toxic among these bring aflatoxin B_1. Aflatoxins B_2, G_1, G_1, M_1 and M_2 are substitution derivations of B_1 and more comparatively less toxic. In terms of occurrence also, B_1 is more preponderent than others. *Aspergillus flavus, Aspergillus parasiticus* and *Aspergillus niger* are known to elaborate aflatoxins under conditions suitable for mould growth.

Detoxification

Aflatoxins, once formed, the difficult to be neutralized by known mild processes. Many kinds of treatments have been examined for detoxification of preformed aflatoxins.

Treatment with a mixture of calcium hydroxide and formaldehyde has shown promise. But this method is impracticable and costly. Simple exposure to fumes of ammonia is the most effective and practical method, used in many western countries. Exposure to sunlight in thin layers for 6-12 hrs has been effective in destroying preformed aflatoxin to a considerable extent.

Infestation of feeds with toxin-producing moulds can occur during many stages: when crop is standing in the field, during harvesting, during drying, during storage etc. The growth of the mould can be arrested by use of fungi-stats in the feed. The common fungi stats used are, cropper sulphate, sodium propionate or propionic acid: gention violet etc. when feed/ingredients are to be stored particularly during inclement weather, addition of any one or a combination of the fungistats would help to arrest fungal multiplication.

Effects in chicks

The primary visible effect of large doses of aflatoxin in young chicks is severe reduction in weight gains, feed intake and feed efficiency. Severe mortality in young chicks is seen from 4 ppm B_1. The effects are dose-related. Mortality ranging from 18 % to 25 % may be seen upto the first 3 weeks of life with levels higher than 4 ppm. It may reach 100 % in unusually high levels of the toxin. Lower levels and survivors show listlessness, ruffled feathering and morbidity.

Postmortem lesions are characteristic. Primary organ affected is liver which is mottled with rounded edges. It is pale yellow in colour and has pin-point heamorrhages. Both size and weight are increased. These can be seen from 1 ppm B_1 onwards.

Spleen is not generally affected

Bursa of fabricius is atrophied and regressed

Kidney is enlarged

Pancreas is unaffected

These changes are prominent at high toxin doses. At lower levels, similar changes occur but with less intensity.

The severity of symptoms and changes in the organs are also influenced by the age of the birds at which toxin is introduced in the feed. Older birds tolerate toxin slightly better than younger birds.

Immunosuppression

A major effect of aflatoxin in animals and birds is break in immunity, even in vaccinated subjects. Toxin-affected birds have frequent relapse of Marek's Ranikhet and other viral infections even after vaccination against those diseases. The mechanism of immunosuppression in the avian species have been studied. Our studies have shown that is the humoral immunity, rather than cell-mediated immunity that operative in aflatoxicosis. Even humoral immunity was adversely affected by aflatoxin with only primary vaccination and was negated by booster vaccination.

Relative toxicity of aflatoxins

The relative toxicity of 4 aflatoxin in ducklings has been presented. The oral LD_{50} dose for each is as follows:

Aflatoxin B1 18.2 g/50 g body weight

Aflatoxin G1 39.2 g/50 g body weight

Aflatoxin B2 84.8 g/50 g body weight

Aflatoxin G2 172.5 g/50 g body weight

Similarly species' differences occur in their susceptibility to aflatoxins. The order of the aflatoxin fractions in decreasing order in potency is as:

$B_1 > G_1 > B_2 > G_2$ for ducklings of the various animals' studies, sheep appear to be most repractory to aflatoxin toxicity and most common symptoms is bile duck hyper placia.

Incidence of aflatoxin infestation of feeds

A sample survey of *Aspergillus* and other fungal infestation was carried out not only by APAU but also by other laboratories in the country. The study showed the *Aspergillus* and other toxin-producing fungi are ubiquitous in distribution. Our results are presented below:

Fungal contaminants

GNC	Rice polish
Aspergillus flavus	*A. flavus*
Aspergillus niger	*A. niger*
Rhizopus spp	*Rhizopus* spp.
Penicillium spp	*Mucour* spp.

Similarly, the occurrence of aflatoxin in various poultry feed ingredients was recorded. Salient data on the above are tabulated below:

		Feedstuffs			
Region	***District***	*GNC*	*Maize*	*Pearl millet*	*Rice polish*
Coastal	Krishna	1.083	0.041	0.042	0.028
	Nellore	0.864	0.082	0.041	0.024
	X	0.974	0.062	0.041	0.026
	Chittore	0.603	0.109	0.032	0.023
Rayalaseema	Kurnool	0.543	0.099	0.035	0.022
Karimnagar	0.229	0.048	0.038	0.019	
Telangana	Ranga Reddy	0.215	0.055	0.043	0.020

Further studies also indicated that among the common feedstuffs in the above region, the ones mostly affected with aflatoxins are: groundnut cake (10/10), pearl millet (6/10) and rice polish (4/10). Broken rice (rice kani) was least affected.

CHAPTER

2

PROGRESS TOWARDS BIOSYNTHETIC RATIONALE OF AFLATOXIN PATHWAYS

Sashidhar Rao, B

Department of Biochemistry University College of Science Osmania University Hyderabad - 500 007

Aflatoxins are potent carcinogenic, mutagenic and toxin secondary metabolites produced by the fungal species, *Aspergillus flavus* link ex. Fries and *A. parasiticus* speare. Aflatoxins have received world-wide attention due to their potentialities as toxic chemical agents entering the food chain, thus posing a threat to human and animal health (1,2). Currently, aflatoxin seems to be an unavoidable environmental contaminant, found naturally occurring in wide range of food and feed consumed by man and farm animals. Presently, it has been recognized, that aflatoxins are of considerable importance from both health and economic angle. The health aspects are based on, (a) the adverse effects of aflatoxin-contaminated feeds on animal health and productivity and (b) the presence of aflatoxins in agricultural commodities and its residue or toxin metabolites in animal tissues meant for human consumption. Enactment of strict legislations governing the presence of aflatoxin in food/ feed (tolerance limit) has resulted in disastrous impact on trade and economy of nations exporting agricultural commodities (3).

Chemically, aflatoxins are biologically active, highly oxygenated heterocyclic compounds (poly-13-ketides), characterised by dihydrodifurano or bis-dihydrodifurano moiety fused toa substituted coumarin molecule. The mutagencity and carcinogencity of aflatoxin are associated with the bisdihydrofurano moiety. Untill, now, about 17 naturally occurring compounds have been discovered, of these aflatoxin B_1, B_2, G_1, and G_2 are the principle metabolites. Aflatoxin B_1 is generally found in the greatest concentration, However, the relative concentration of other principle metabolites varies depending on the fungal strain, substrate and condition of growth. Three most important factors controlling aflatoxin formation in agricultural commodities are relative humidity, moisture and temperature.

In view of the above considerations, it is implicit, that he scientific research be oriented towards the prevention of aflatoxin formation. This goal can be achieved only with proper understanding of the biochemical pathway leading to aflatoxin biogenesis and various factors involved in its formation. Investigations carried out during the last two decades, has led to the elucidation of the metabolic pathway of aflatoxin formation (4,5).

AFLATOXIN- SECONDARY METABOLITE PAR EXCELLENCE:

Broadly, the biochemical processes occurring in a living fungal cell can be divided into three categories, namely the basal metabolism, replicatory process and secondary metabolism. Basal metabolism and replicatory process constitutes the primary metabolism, and involves the anabolic and catabolic reactions. The products formed during primary metabolism are essential for life. Secondary metabolism stems from the primary metabolism, and on the other hand, it is not indispensable in cellular metabolism. In general, the secondary metabolities or idiolites are not involved in growth and often synthesized after growth has ceased. Enzymes involved in secondary metabolism are active or formed at the commencement and during the idiophase of growth (6). Idiolites are produced typically as members of a particular chemical family because of the low specificity of some enzymes involved in secondary metabolism.

Aflatoxins are idealities, largely produced by anabolic route, and their synthesis consumes energy and reducing power generated from primary metabolism. Earlier, elucidation of the mechanism of aflatoxin biosynthesis was centered on establishment of intermediates in the pathway. During the past two decades, many intermediates involved in the formation of aflatoxin B_1 have been identified (4,5) Fig.1 gives the outline of the metabolic pathway leading in the formation aflatoxin B_1 from acetate. Some of the important enzymes involved in the biogenesis of aflatoxin B_1 has been listed in table 1. Even though, there is a general agreement on the identity of the intermediates and enzymes involved in aflatoxin B_1biosynthesis, there is much to be learned with respect to the enzymology of the process involved. Much of the present knowledge on aflatoxin biogenesis is based on the putative precursors isotopically labeled with ^{14}C, ^{3}H, ^{13}C, ^{18}O, followed by NMR spectroscopy. The identities and sequence of production of several intermediates were determined by using blocked mutants (auxotropic mutants), metabolic inhibitors and radioactive labeling with resting cells and cell-free extracts of Aspergillus ssp. Only few enzymes involved in the aflatoxin biosynthesis have been purified or extensively characterized (5,7). The metabolic inter-relationship between aflatoxins (B_2, G_1, B_1) is unclear. Earlier, it was postulated that, aflatoxin B_2, G_1, B_2 are derived from aflatoxin B1. However, recent investigations have shown that, there is no inter-conversion of aflatoxin B_1 to B_2, G_1, G_2 by intact cell of blocked mutants of *A. parasiticus* (8). In the recent past, newer approaches, such as, application of fungal protoplast system are being used to localize enzymatic system involved in aflatoxin production and their regulation (9).

The rationale behind, effective prevention of aflatoxin formation in agricultural commodities, involved proper understanding of aflatoxin biogenesis and its regulation. It is now becoming clear that newer powerful techniques, such as r-DNA technique, immunohistochemistry, and NMR spectroscopy of cells, will have to be applied. As a novel approach, would it be possible to alter the genes that make the enzymes, which are responsible for toxin formation ?

REFERENCES

1. Mycotoxins 1987. Report on the second Joint FAO/WHO/UNEP international conference on mycotoxins held in Bangkok, Thailand, Food and Agricultural Organization, Rome. 1988.
2. Global Environmental Monitoring System. Assessment of chemical contamination in food. Report on the results of the UNEP/FAO/WHO programme on health-related environmental monitoring. 1988.
3. Aflatoxins: Research, Analysis and Control. JAOCS. 66: 1398-1413: 1989.
4. Steyn, P.S. (Ed). The biosynthesis of Mycotoxins: A Study in Secondary Metabolism. P105-155; Academic Press, New York, London. Toranto, 1980.
5. Dutton, M.F. Enzymes of Aflatoxin Biosynthesis. Microbiol. Rev. 52 : 274-295: 1988.
6. Demain, A.L. Regulation of Secondary Metabolism in Fungi. Pure, Appl. Chem. 58 : 219-226 : 1986.
7. Bhatnagar, D. Ullah, H.J. and Cleveland, T.E. Purification and Characterization of Methyltransferase from *Aspergillus parasitius* SRRC 163 involved in Aflatoxin Biosynthetic pathway. Prep. Biochem. 14 : 321-349 : 1988.

8. Bhatnagar, D., McCormic, S.R. Lee, L.S. and Hill, R.A. Identification of O-methylsterigmatocystin as a Aflatoxin B1 and G1 precursor in *Aspergillus parastitucus.* Appl. Environ, Microbiol. 53 : 1028-1037 : 1987.

9. Peberdy, J.F. and Ferenczy, L. Fungal Protoplasts: Applications in Biochemistry and Genetics. Vol. 6 p189-203. Marcel Dekker Inc. New York and Basel, 1985.

FIG- 1

PROPOSED BIOGENESIS OF AFLATOXINS

ACETATE 1, 2, 3, 4, 5

↓

NORSOLORINIC ACID

↓ 6

AVERANTIN

↓ 7,8

AVERUFIN

↓ 9, 10

VERSICONAL HEMIACTEAL ACETATE

↓ 11, 12, 13

VERSICOLORIN A

↓ 14, 15, 16, 17, 18, 19

STERIGNATOCYSTIN

↓ 19, 20

O- METHYLSTERIGATOCYSTIN

↓ 21

AFLATOXIN B1

*1-21 ARE THE ENZYMES INVOLVED IN THE METABOLIC PATHWAY (REFER, TABLE-1 FOR DETAILS).

TABLE -1 ENZYMES INVOLVED IN THE BIOSYNTHESIS OF AFLATOXIN

ENZYMES	ORDER OF ENZYME ACTION	PRODUCT OF ENZYME ACTION
Acetyl CoA carboxylase (E)*	1	Malonyl CoA
Acetyltransferase (E)	2	Primed synthase
Malonyltransferase (E)	3	Primed synthase
Hexamalonyltransferase (I)**	4	Primed synthase
Norsolorinic acid synthase complex (I)	5	Norsolorinic acid anthrone
Norsolorinic acid dehydrogenase (E)***	6	Averantin
Averantin-5'-hydroxylase (H)	7	5'-hydroxy-Averantin
5'-hydroxy-Averantin dehydrogenase (I)	8	Averufin
Versicoloronal synthase (H)	10	Versiconal-acetate
Versiconal acetate hydrolase (E)	11	Versicolorin B
Versicolorin B oxidase (H)	12	Versicolor-hemiacetal
Versicolor hemiacetal-dehydratase (H)	13	Versicolor
Versicolor reductase (H)	14	6-deoxy-versicolor
Versicolor oxygenase (H)	15	Versicolor-lactone
lactonase (I)	16	THBCA
THBCA decarboxylase (I)	17	THB
Methyltransferase (I)	18	THMB
Xanthone Cyclase (I)	19	Sterigmatocystin
Methyltransfterase (E)	20	Sterigmatocystin
Oxide-reductase (E)	21	Aflatoxin B1

TJNCA. trihydroxybenzophenone-6'-carboxylic acid; THMB, trihydroxy-6-methoxy-benzophenone; THB, tetrahydroxybenzophenone. * (E)-Enzyme identified: (I) ** Enzyme inferred from similar system; *** (H) - Hypothetical enzymes.

CHAPTER

3 IMPORTANT LESSER KNOWN TOXIC FUNGI IN FEED- AN UPDATE

M.A. Sattar,
All India Coordinated Research Project on Seed Borne Disease,
Rajendranagar, Hyderabad- 500 030.

Fungi are known for producing mycotoxins in the grains even before the corp is harvested. In sorghum, mycotoxin was observed at premature and late stage of the crop (Reddy and Nusrath 1986). Incidence of aflatoxin in Bihar at preharvested stage on *Brassica compestris* (yellow seed sarson) was recorded by Sinha *et al.* (1988). Among the 96 isolates of *aspergillus flavus.* 49 were toxigenic. All the four aflatoxins viz., B_1, B_2, G_2 were produced by *B. Juncea* (brown seeded rai), here also in the 85 isolates of *A. flavus* 49 were toxigenic. Lewellyn *et al.* (1981) found mustard seeds to be of intermediate category for production of aflatoxins. Sinha *et al.* (1988) reported that most of the samples in the marketed wheat were having aflatoxin levels exceeding 20 ppb of safe limit. It has been noted by Punam Kumari *et al.* (1987) in mung bean seeds *Aspergillus flavus* dominated with maximum frequency of 40% samples with aflatoxins and concentration of aflatoxin B_1 was upto 2800 ppb. Out of 124 isolates of *A. flavus* 46 produced aflatoxin. Forty-three isolates produced only aflatoxin B_1 by more than 20 ppb the tolerance level fixed by WHO. Vinod *et al.* (1987) have observed that aflatoxin B_1 formed on maize grains under favourable conditions. At Banswada, Durgapur District of Rajasthan and Panchmahal district of Gujarat experienced an outbreak of hepatitis affecting man and dog, which was due to consumption of spoiled grains. Of the various mycotoxins, only aflatoxins have attracted the great attention all over the world (Wagon, 1965 and Anon., 1977).

Paul Neergaard (1979) has reported the following fungi-producing mytoxins in the field and during storage in the grains: *Aspergillus flavus. A parasiticus* (aflatoxin complex). *A. candidus, A. fumigatus* and *A. ochracus* (Ochratoxin complex). *Pencilium islandicum* (islanditoxin). *P. citrinum* (citinin). *P. rubrum* (rubratoxin), *P. viridicatum* (hepatoxin and nephrotoxic). It has been reported that some species of *Aspergillus oryzae, A niger, A. wentii* and *A. ruber* aflatoxin but Pandey *et al.* (1989) confirmed that two species of *A. flavus* and *A. parasiticus* produce aflatoxin. Besides aflatoxin, cyclopiazonic acid and sterigmatocystin are also toxin products of *A. flavus.* Cyclopinzonic acid is an idole tartaric acid which was isolated from *Pencillium cyuclopium* and *A. versicolor.* Toxicity of this in poultry causes change in posture due to the rigid extension of legs following death. It is interesting to note that grains appearing healthy without any moulds at all may be highly toxic and not all the isolates are toxic.

In Kumaun hills and tarai areas of Naini Tal, from different substrate, 300 isolates of *A. flavus* and 70 isolates of *A parasiticus* were isolated by Pandey *et al.* (1989). Out of 300 isolates of *A. flavus* 66.6% produced aflatoxins, 83.3% of the total aflatoxigenic and non-aflatoxigenic strains produced cyclopiazonic acid and only 8.66% strains produced sterigmatocystin. Cyclopiazonic acid contamination may be more common and widespread in food and feed. High percentage of aflatoxin producers have loas yielded cyclopiazonic acid. 120 isolates of *Aspergillus flavus* produced both aflatoxin and cyclopiazonic acid. In the same study the other 130 isolates produced cyclopiazonic acid and 80 isolates yielded aflatoxin alone. A few strains of *A. flavus* produced all the four aflatoxin (B_1, B_2, G_1 and G_2). Aflatoxin B_2 and found in each and every toxigenic strain of *A. flavus* isolates from any of the substrate (cereal grains, spices. dry fruits, soil, pulses, vegetable, air contamination, cheese and bread). All the 70 isolates of *A. purasiticus* produced though in few of the strain potential was very low (12 ug/b), amount of aflatoxin varies in different isolates of *A. parasiticus.* Higher percentage (100) of potential toxigenic strains was noted in *A. parasiticus* when compared to *A. flavus.* In one of the isolates of *A. flavus* from solid of poultry farm in Haldwani, production of aflatoxin (B_1 only) was very high 139/1 as compared to other strains of *A. flavus.* Thus, now there is a need for the consideration of cyclopiazonic acid. In the studies of aflatoxin producing potential, Reddy (1987) observed that out of 54 isolates of *A. flavus* only 18 (35%) were toxigenic. 13 produced aflatoxin B_1, isolates 8 and 4 produced aflatoxin B_2 and G_1 respectively. He described the fungi-producing toxins @ 7200 ug/ml as highly toxigenic. 50 to 200 ug as moderately toxigenic and /50 ug/ml as less toxigenic.

Toxin production

This depends on the species or strains and the ecological condition for its development, in particular source, temperature and humidity. In England during 1960, one-lakh turkey poults died from feed in which one for the constituents was groundnut invaded by *A. flavus*. The fungus may produce the toxin on different grains in varying quantities but most strains from tropical and subtropical regions produce aflatoxin. Highest amount of aflatoxin is produced in groundnut, wheat and rice, it is also produced in cotton seed, soybeans and maize.

For the growth of *A. flavus* and production of mycotoxin minimum of about 85% relative humidity is required. Mycelial growth takes in the wide range from 6 to 46°C, but aflatoxin is produced between 13-41°C, optimum being 28°C.

When *A. niger* or *Rhizoctonia solani* is present, *A. flavus* produces less aflatoxin and there may be other such microbial interactions.

A. flavus becomes dominent, especially when shells are damaged before harvest: kernels are exposed to infection leading to production of aflatoxin. Delayed harvest and post-harvest drying conditions increase toxin production.

Impact of fungi on animal health

Pathogenic fungi cause many diseases in animals, some by direct effect, other by consumption of food made toxic by fungi. It is due to (i) accumulation of the pathogen in a limited space, spores are disbursed during harvest of contaminated crop, (ii) development of increased sensitivity by continuous exposure to high concentration of pathogenic agents and (iii) grains, and other stuff containing toxic metabolities which are not detectable by ordinary visual inspection.

Mycotoxicosis is caused due to mycotoxins which are produced by field and storage fungi. In the case of egotism, poisoning takes place due to alkaloids in the selerotia of *Claviceps purpura* is known from ancient times as a cause of St. Anthony's Fire of middle Ages. Cattle, a sheep and poultry are sensitive to poison and ergot flour consiption has caused death. Toxins from *Claviceps paspali* causes damage to the nervous system. Fusaritoxicosis is caused due to the toxins produced by various species of *Fusarium*. It has been observed that toxins produced by *f. nivale* causes vomiting, *F. sporotrichoides* causes bone marrow exhaustion. This toxin is produced in various cereals in particular millets and maximum production takes place at 0-5°C. Diarhoea and loss of weight has been observed by toxins produced by *F. equiseti (F. scirpi)* and *F. tricinctum*. Zearalenone called F2 produced by *F. graminearum*. *F. moniliforme*, *F. oxysporium* and

F. tricinctum causes oestrogen syndromes or hyperestrogenism results in infertility in swan and dairy cattle. The toxicity of natural products from *Fusarium* is of greater incidence and perhaps more important than aflatoxin.

Aflatoxicosis

Most common being aflatoxin B_1, B_2, G_1 and G_2 produced by *Aspergillus flavus. A parasitucus.* In poultry, especially young turkeys and ducks. Turkey 'X' disease was very popular. The disease develops inappetence, poor growth rate, subcutaenous haemorrhage of the legs, feet and back, a staggering gait and sudden death is observed. Livers from these birds were found to be enlarged. Characteristic effect is liver damage. It is by proliferation of the bile ducts, fibrosis and necrosis: haemorrhages occur in the internal tracts and degenerative changes in the kidneys are observed. After prolong intake of sublethal amounts malignant liver tumours develop in some animals. Aflatoxin B is regarded as the most active hepatocarcinogen known. In regions of Africa where groundnut, often highly contaminated with aflatoxin, is largely consumed as an important source of protein, the frequency of liver cancer is about 100 times higher than in Europe.

Nephrotoxicosis

These mycotoxins are produced by different species of *Aspergillus* and *Pencillium,* the ocratoxin complex by *A. ochraceus,* citrin by *P. viridicatum, P. citrinum, P. expansum* and other species of *Penillium* Citrinin is found in nature in 'yellowed-rice' invaded by fungi of this group. *P. viriducatum* appears to be the main producer of citrinin in cereals.

Mould nephrosis or porcine nephropathy is known to be associated with feeding of mouldy grains in Denmark. This toxin causes depression of growth rate and increased water consumption and diaresis, chronic damage of the kidney in the form of tubular cells, formation of connective tissues and cyst.

The rubratoxins from *P. rubrum* caused liver damage and disseminated haemorrhage in horse, cattle, pig, dog and chicken. In the laboratory studies luteoskyrin from *P islandicum* was found to cause liver damage similar to that caused by aflatoxin.

Nerurotoxicosis

Citreoviridina metabolic product of *P. citreo- viride,* causes damage of central nervous system resulting in progressive paralysis and respiratory failure in pigeon etc.

Aspergillosis caused by species of *Aspergillus* is most important which is common in birds. Main cause is *A. fumigatus,* a common storage fungi in grain. This affects pulmonary tissues. It is mostly observed in newly-hatched fowls, mycelium covers the lungs and spores make the breathing impossible. In chicken and turkeys, it caused panophthalmitis (general inflamation of the eye ball) and fungus grows luxuriantly in the vitreous body.

For the control of fungi in grains the following are the findings:

1. Sorghum crop should be harvested around 40 days from mean date of anthesis as highest level of germination.
2 Preharvest rains at 25-30 days after flowing of paddy adversely affects of storability – so such seed should be avoided.
3. The moisture content just before storage should not be more than .9, 10, 9 and 6 per cent, for paddy, jawar, green gram and maize, respectively.
4. Storage in dry place.

Studies carried out to attempt the control measures are presented below:

Premlata Singh *et al.* (1987) reported that earlier various chemicals have been shown to destroy aflatoxins in naturally-contaminated materials viz., chlorine, ozone, hydrochloric acid, benzoyl peroxide, ammonia, sodium hydroxide and ethanolamine. They observed that common salt (NaCl) @ 500 ppm completely inhibited the production of aflatoxin B_2, whereas aflatoxin B_1 was inhibited only 64 to 74.2% in different concentrations i.e. 500 to 10,000 ppm respectively. One of the control measures is to have resistant grains. For this, Reddy (1987a) screened sorghum cultivator for aflatoxin production. Antiaflatoxin properties of some plant extracts were observed by Reddy (1987b) and he observed that paddy seeds treated with the extracts of 20 plants and subsequently inoculated with toxigenic strains of *Aspergilus flavus,* had a pronounced inhibitory effect on the production of aflatoxin-B_1. Maximum inhibition (65%) of aflatoxin B_1 was with the leaves and stem extracts of *Ricinus communis.* Use of such non-toxic agents to control the growth of grain-destroying moulds and mycotoxin production is always preferable.

REFERENCES

Anonymous. 1977. Report of the Joint FAO/WHO/UNDP Conference on mycotoxins, 19-27. Sept. Nairobi, Kenya.

Anonymous. 1990. Work directly useful to farmers. Seed Technology Research Project, Rajendranagar, Hyderabad.

Hanza Pandey, Jyoti Saxena, Neeta Pande, S.K. Pande and B.S. Mehrotra. 1989. Screening of various substrates for mycotoxin-producing potential of *Aspergillus flavus* and *A. parasiticus.* Indian Phytopath. **42**: 132-136.

Neergaard, Paul. 1979. Seed pathology, Vol. I, pp 839. Macmillan Press Ltd., London and Tokyo.

Premlata Singh, Syed Khalid Ahmed and Sita Bhagat. 1987. Effect of salinity on aflatoxin production by *Aspergillus flavus.* Indian Phytopath. **40:** 553-555.

Punam Kumari and K.K. Sinha. 1987. Aflatoxin elaboration in Mung bean seeds. Indian Phytopath. **40:** 201-203.

Reddy, B.N. and Nusrath, M. 1986. Stage of sorghum in the field susceptible to fungal invasion and mycotoxin formation. Indian Phytopath. **39:** 106-110.

Reddy, B.N. 1987. Screening of sorghum cultivars for aflatoxin production. Indian Phytopath. **40:** 549-550.

Reddy, B.N. 1987b. Aflatoxin-producing potential of *Aspergillus flavus* isolate from sorghum. Indian Phytopath. **40:** 550-551.

Reddy, B.N. 1987c. Anti-aflatoxin properties of some plant extracts. Indian Phytopath. **40** : 551-552.

Sinha, A.K., K.S., Bilgrami, K.S. Ranjan and T. Prasad. 1988. Incidence of aflatoxin and mustard crop in Bihar, Indian Phytopath. **41:** 434-437.

Sinha, K.K. and A.K. Sinha, 1988. Occurrence of aflatoxin and *Aspergillus flavus* in marketed wheat. Indian Phytopath. **41:** 44-47.

Vinod, K. Gaur and Babu Singh Siradhana. 1987. Indian Phytopath. **40:** 430-437.

CHAPTER

4 OCHRATOXIN A IN BIOLOGICAL SYSTEMS AND ITS ANALYSIS

S.M. Reddy
Department of Botany,
Kakatiya University, Warangal - 506 009.

Ochratoxins are first major group of toxins discovered after aflatoxins. Vander Merwe *et al.* (1965). were the first to characterise Ochratoxin A and B. Ochratoxins are a group of seven isocoumarin derivatives linked with an amide bond to the amino group of L-B-phe-nylalanine. Ochratoxin A is a 7-carboxy-5-chloro-8-hydroxy-3, 4 di-dydro-3R-methylisocoumarin which is linked through the carboxyl group to L-phenylalanine.

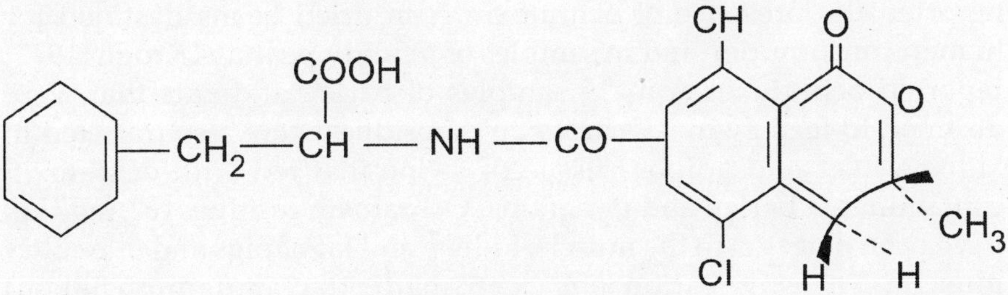

OCHRATOXIN A

Ochratoxin A is the predominant and most toxin member of the series and majority of the literature has been concerned with this mycotoxin. Ochratoxin A and its methyl and /ethyl (ochratoxin C) esters were approximately equitoxic and were considerable more potent than ochratoxin B. Ochratoxin B was essentially non-toxic. The presence of chlorine atom ochratoxin A has been considered a primary determinant of toxicity of these compounds.

Ochratoxin A is a colourless cyrstalline compound which is highly soluble in polar organic solvents. Slightly soluble in water and dissolves in aqueous sodium hydrogen carbonate.

Organisms producing ochratoxins:

Scott (1965) first isolated ochratoxin A from *Aspergillus ochraceus*

(K-804) isolated from sorghum grains. At present a total of 1 species of *Aspergillus (A. sulphreus, A. sclerotiorum, A. alliaceus, A, melleus, A. ochraceous, A. ostinus and A. petrakii)* are reported to elaborate this toxin. Similarly after the report of production of this toxin by *Penicillium viridicatum* by Van Walbeck *et al.* (1969) *P. palitans, P. commune, P. purpurscens, P. verruculosum, P. variable* and *P. cyclopium* were also reported to produce ochratoxins. However, *A. ochraceus* and *P. viriducatum* are leading producers under natural conditions.

Natural occurence:

Shotwell *et al.* (1969) first reported its natural occurrence in corn. Subsequently Scott *et al.* (1970) reported it on Canadian wheat. It is now a known natural contaminant of various agricultural commodities from more than 10 countries (table 1).

Barley appears to be most common commodity of contamination of ochratoxins producing organisms. Reiss (1978, 1981) reported the occurrence of *A. ochraceus* in cake and bread. Scott *et al.* (1972) reported the presence of ochratoxin A in dried beans destined for human consumption and in samples of mouldy peanuts. Krogh (1972) reported ochratoxin A in 19 samples of barley and oats that were destined to feed swine. Ochratoxin A residues were also detected in kidney, liver and adipose tissue of swine that fed with ochratoxin contaminated barley and oat grains. Ochratoxin residues (67 mg/kg) have been detected in the muscle, kidney and fat of pigs and in poultry muscle. The suggestion has been made that endemic (Baken) nephropathy, a human disease of unknown etiology reported from Bulgaria, Rumania and Yugoslavia may be associated with elevated ochratoxin A. The above findings indicate that human exposure to ochratoxin A may occur not only through consumption of mouldy plant materials but also through consumption of animal products.

Factors influencing ochratoxin production:

Ochratoxin production by either *A. ochraceus* or *P. viridicatum* is mainly influenced by two factors such as water activity (a_w) and temperature. Northolt (1979) determined the influence of temperature and water activity on achratoxin production by *A ochraceus.* A minimum temperature at which ochratoxin production was noticed at 4°C for *P. viridicatum* and 12°C for *A. ochraceus* and optimum temperature recorded for its production was 18°C. *P. viridicatum* is reported to grow over a temperature range of 4°C-30°C and optimum was 20°C. Similarly *A. ochraceus* becomes dominant in corn stored for

Table 1: Natural occurrence of Ochratoxin A in foods and feeds of Plant origin

Commodity	Country	No. of samples analysed	Percentage of contaminated	Ochratoxin A level (range, mg/kg)
Foods:				
Maize	USA	293	1.0	83-166
Maize	France	463	2.6	15-200
Maize	India	21	-	30-50
Maize	Yogoslavia	191	25.7	45-5215
Wheat	USA	286	2.8	5-115
Wheat	Canada	4	1.0	20-100
Wheat	India	24	8.0	30-50
Barley	Denmark	50	6.0	9-189
Barley	USA	182	12.6	10-29
Barley	Yugoslavia	64	12.4	14-27
Barley	Czechoslovakia	48	2.1	3800
Barley	Sweden	269	6.3	2-20
Sorghum	India	24	12.5	50-70
Groundnut	India	18	11.0	50-200
Ragi	India	15	-	70
Rice	Japan	2	100.0	230-430
Bread	UK	50	2.0	210
Flour	UK	7	28.5	490-2900
Beans	Sweden	71	8.5	10-442
Coffee Beans	USA	267	7.1	22-360
Peas	Sweden	72	2.8	10-15
Barley, Oats	Denmark	33	57.6	28-27500
Feeds:				
Barley, Wheat oats, rye, maize	Poland	150	5.3	50-200
Mixed feed	Poland	203	4.9	10-50
Maize feed	Yugoslavia	191	25.7	45-5125
Barley, oats	Sweden	84	8.3	16-409
Wheat, hay	Canada	95	7.4	30-6000
Wheat, oats, barley, rye	Canada	32	56.3	30-27000

several weeks at 25°C and 18.5% moisture (Lopez and Christension, 1967).

Raulin-Thom and YES medium were used for production of ochratoxin by *A. ochraceus* and *P. viridicatum*. Addition of phenylalanine (1% greatly stimulated ochratoxin production. Similarly combined addition of trace elements Fe, Zn, Cu, Bo, Mn and Mo increased the synthesis of ochratoxin A synthesis (Ferreria, 1968). Northolt (1979) determined that a minimum water activity (aw) required for production of ochratoxin A was 0.83-0.87 Isolation and preparative purification of the ochratoxin:

Three extraction techniques are used for solid samples.

a) Soxhlet extraction

b) Blending with a solvent in a waring blender for 1-3 min.

c) Shaking of the solid for 10-30 min. with the solvent.

The following solvents are in use for extraction of ochratoxin A.

1. Chloroform: methanol (1:1)
2. Methanol: water: hexane (55: 45: 40)
3. Methanol: water: hexane (55: 40: 40) + 1% H_2SO_4 (20%)
4. Chloroform: methanol: hexane (8: 2: 1)
5. Chloroform: water (4% Kill) (9:1)
6. Chloroform: methanol (7:3)
7. Acetonitrile: water: hexane (9:1:5)

Vander Merwe *et al.* (1965) extracted the ochratoxin A, B from the crude extract (in chloroform) with aqueous $NaHCO_3$. The ochratoxins are obtained from the aqueous layer by acidification and extraction into chloroform.

At present the crude extract is partitioned between hexane, 85% methanol followed by combination of the methanolic layer in vacuum and partition between chloroform and water

The ochractoxin A and B are obtained from the organic layer by extraction with $NaHCO_3$ acidification and extraction into chloroform.

Ochratoxin containing mixtures can also be separated on formamide impregnated cellulose powder and elution with mixture of hexane and benzene.

Scott *et al.* (1971) reported that ochratoxin A was eluted from silica gel, oxalic acid (95:5 by elution with chloroform: acetone (99:1 or 98:2) and applied methodology of the large scale preparation of ochratoxin A. Peterson and Ciegler (1978) reported the purification of ochratoxin A using liquid-liquid extractions and final cleanup up preparative HPLC.

Fermented wheat (2.274 kg)

↓

Grind in Waring blender with equal weight of water

↓

Extract twice with methanol

↓

Methanol solution (18,500 ml, 6.13 g of OTA)

↓

Add NaCl (3M) extract twice with methylene chloride

↓

Methylene chloride solution (3,760 ml, 3.76 g of OTA) Extract with 0.2 M $NaHCO_3$

↓

Hydrogen carbonate solution (acidify to pH 2.5 with con, HCl)

Extract with chloroform

↓

Methylene chloride solution (1750 ml, 3.5 g OTA)

↓

Filter through (Na_2SO_4 Evaporate to dryness at room temperature

↓

Ethyl acetate solution, filter and evaporate to dryness

↓

Ethyl acetate solution (32 ml, 7.2 OTA) inject into HPLC

↓

Evaporate active fraction to dryness

↓

Crystalize OTA from benezene.

TLC determination of Ochratoxin A in food stuffs: *

(Schematic representation of procedure)

Extract 50g of sample its 25 ml 0.1 mol/1H_3PO_4 + 250 ml chloroform

↓

Filter through whatman No.1 filter paper

↓

Collect 50 ml filtrate

↓

Partition 50 ml of filtrate on sodium bicarnonate-celite column (retain remainder for confirmation of identity)

↓

Wash column with 70 ml chexane

↓

Wash column with 70 ml chloroform

↓

Elute ochratoxin A with 100 ml acetic acid: Benezene (5:95)

↓

Evaporate eluate to near dryness

↓

Transfer eluate to 8 ml vial with acetic acid: benzene (1:99)

↓

Evaporate extract to dryness

↓

Dissolve extract in 0.5 ml acetic acid: benzene (1:99)

↓

Separate by Silica gel TLC; mobile phase, benzene, acetic acid: methanol (90:5:5)

↓

Quantity by visual or densitometric comparision under long-wave UV.

* (Environmental carcinogens Selected methods of Analysis, Editor-in chief, H. Egan, TARC publication No. 44, France, pp2 225-270, 1982)

HPLC determination of ochratoxins A in food stuffs*

(Schematic representation of procedure)

Extract 60g of sample in blender with 25 ml 0.1 mol/1 H_3PO_4 and 250 ml of ethyl acetate

↓

Filter through fluted filter paper, collect 180 ml

↓

Extract ochratoxin A from ethyl acetate with 3 x 25 ml 3% sodium bicarbonate

↓

Acidify to pH 3 with 1 mol/1 HCL and extract with 2 x 50 ml ethyl acetate

↓

Pass through Na_2SO_4 to remove water and evaporate to dryness

↓

Chromatograph on 50 silica gel 60

↓

Elute column with 0.2% methylene chloride: methanol: acetic acid (97:3:0.2)

↓

Evaporate eluate to near dryness

↓

Divide extract into 2 equal parts

↓

Prepare HPLC standard curve in range 5,10, 20, 40, 80 ng ochratoxin A, each injected in the same volume (25ul) on reversed phase column using mobile phase of KH_2PO_4 (0.01 ml/1) in water:acetonitrile (45:55)

↓

Determine ochratoxin A in simple from standard curve.

*(Environmental Carcinogens Selected Methods of Analysis, Editor-in-chief H. Egan, IARC publication No. 44, France, pp 271-282.)

Biological activity of Ochratoxin A

Zebra fish and brine shrimp leave were sensitive on ochratoxin A (Abedi and Scott, 1969). Most of the bacteria were insensitive (Arai and Otomo, 1969), while actinomycetes were inhibited at the conc. of 100-500 mg/ml (Arai and Otomo, 1969). Ochratoxin exhibited cytotoxicity to Hela cells. It also induced mitotic abnormalities in monkey epithelial cell tissue culture cells (Broce *et al.* 1970). Ochratoxin at 100 mg/30 ducklings caused liver changes characterised by swelling and structural damage of mitochondria, morphological changes in the endoplasmic reticulum and fatty infiltration of hepatocytes (Theron *et al.* 1966).

Ochratoxin at 100 mg developed a focal areas of liver cell necrosis and hyaline degeneration in rats. Proliferation of smooth ER with formation of masses of SM within the liver cell cytoplasm referred to as finger prints. Ochratoxin A at LD 50 value of 20-22 mg/kg induced necrossis of the renal tubules and periportal cells of the liver. Glycogen accumulation was observed in liver cells. On oral feeding for 90 days at 0.2 ppm concentration developed distal convoluted tubules of kidney cells.

Ochratoxin at 166 to 216 μg/chick affected the chick by causing diarrhoea and haemarrhage in the liver, kidneys and proventricules. Sublethal doses of ochratoxin A produced does related growth depression. Birds dying after administration of the toxin had visceral gout and acute nephrosis. Hepatic lesions occurred less often than renal lesions and included mild, diffused vacuolisation of hepatosis and foci of necrosis. Surviving and dead birds showed suppression of haemoisis in the bone marrow and depletion of the lymphoid elements from the spleen and bursa of Fabricius. The birds also suffered entritis. Laying hens fed diets at 2 or 4 ppm levels for six months showed 1864% mortality respectively. Growth depression was also noted in male broiler chicks fed diets containing ochratoxi A. A dose dependent increase in relative weight ofthe crop, pancreas, liver and gizzard and significant regression of the bursa Faricicius was recorded. Experimental feeding of graded levels of cohratoxin A in diets has a detrimental effect on growing chicks (Prior *et al.* 1980; Kubena *et al.* 1985). A drastic decrease in total proteins, albumin, cholesterol and aspartate amino transferase activity was reported by Kubena *et al.* (1988) in growing broiler chicks fed with ochratoxin A.

Ochratoxin A was detectable in blood and liver, excretes in urine and faeces over a 72 hour period (Purchase and Nel, 1967). Two other compounds ochratoxin α and 4-hydroxy ochratoxin formed due to the loss of phenylalanine from Ochratoxin A were also present in the loss of phenylalanine from Ochratoxin A were also present in the urine. These hydrolytic activities in the rat was predominantly localised in small intestine preparation with significantly lesser amounts found in large intestive and liver. Ochratoxin A was detected in decreasing order in liver, kidneys, muscle and placenta of pregnant pigs fed for 8 days. Ochratoxin A and B were also present in the serum but only ochratoxin A was excreted in urine and faeces.

Purchase and Theron (1968) have reported degenerative changes in the rat liver mitochondria including dilation at 10 mg/kg of ochratoxin A. Intramitochondrial ATP pool was rapidly depleted by 80% within 2 min. of treatment with 18 n nol. Ochratoxin a/mg protein. Higher toxin levels produced the total ATP depletion. Ochratoxin A was strongly nephrotoxic to dogs (Szezech *et al.* 1972).

REFERENCES

Abedi, Z.H. and P.M. Scott. *J. Assoc. Off. Anal. Chem.* 52, 1968, 693.

Arai, T. and M.Otomo. *Ann. Rept. Inst. Food. Microbiol. Chiba, Univ.* 22, 1969, 81.

Broce, D., R.M. Grodner, R.L. Killerbrew and F.L. Bonner. *J. Assoc. Off Anal. Chem.* 53, 1970, 616.

Ferreira, N.P.*Antonie Van Leeuwenhoek J. Microbiol. Serol. 34, 1968,* 433.

Krogh, P. Symp. Inter. Union of Pure and Applied Chemistry, Aug. 21-22, 1972, Kungalv, Sweden, (Abstract)

Kubena, L.F., R.B. Harvey, O.J. Flatcher, T.D. Philliops, H.H. Mollenhauer, D.A. Witzel and N.D. Heidelhauch.*Poultry Sci. 64,* 1985, 620.

Lopez, L.C. and C.M. Christensen, *Phytopathology, 57,* 1967, 588.

Peterson, R.E. and A. Liegler, Appl. Environ. Microbiol. 36, 1978, 613.

Prior, M.G., J.B.O. Neill and C.S. Sisodia, *Poultry Sci. 59,* 1980, 1254.

Purchase, I.F.H. and W. Nel. Recent advances in research on ochratoxin. Part I Toxicological aspects in R.T. Mateles and G.N. Wogan (Eds.) Biochemistry of some food-borne microbial toxins. M.I.T. Cambridge, Mass, 1967, pp 153.

Purchase, I.F.H. and J.J. Theron. *Food. Cosmet. Toxicol. 6,* 1968, 479.

Northolt, M.D., H.P. Van Egmond and W.E.Paulsch. *J. Food. Protec.* 42, 1979, 485.

Reiss, J.Z. *Lebensm,-Unters-Forsch. 167,* 1978, 419.

Reiss, J.Deut, Lebensm- Rundsch, 77, 1981, 27.

Scott, De. B. *Mycopathol. Mycol. Appl. 25,* 1965, 213.

Scott, P.M., W.Van. Walbeck, J. Harwig and O.I. Fennel. *Can. J. Pan. 50,* 1970, 583.

Scott, P.M., W. Van Walbeck, B. Kennedy and D. Angeti. *J. Agric. Food. Chem. 20,* 1972, 1103.

Scott, P.M., B. Kennedy and W.Van Walbeck. *J. Assoc. Off. Anal. Chem. 54,* 1971, 1445.

Shotwell, O.L., C.W. Heseltine and M.L. Goulden, *Appl. Microbiol.17,* 1969, 765.

Szezach, G.M., W.W. Carlton and J. Tuite, *Lab. Invest. 26, 1972, 492* Abstract)

Theron, J.J., K.J. Vander Merwe, N.Liebenberg, H. J.B. Joubert and W.Nel. *J. Pathol. Bacteriol. 91,* 1966, 521.

Vander Merwe, K.J., P.S. Steyn and L. Fourie, *J. Chem. Sci.,* 1965, 7083.

Van Walbeck. W., P.M. Scott, J. Harwig and J. W. Lawrence, *Can. J. Microbiol. 15,* 1969, 1281.

CHAPTER

5 GENETIC DIFFERENCES FOR SUSCEPTIBILITY OF AFLATOXINS IN POULTRY

S.C. Mohapatra,
Project Directorate on Poultry,
Rajendranagar, Hyderabad- 500 030.

INTRODUCTION

The Aflatoxins are the toxin substances produced by fungi, mainly *Aspergillus flavus* and *Aspergillus parasiticus.* Among the four different types of aflatoxins (B_1, B_2, G_1 and G_2) and B_1 is the most toxic to poultry and livestock including human beings. The metabolites of the aflatoxin B_1 is presented below. The metabolite M_1 which is excreted in the milk is of special significance to infants and young animals. The metabolite AFB_{2a} is the most toxic as it causes inhibition of enzyme, necrosis of liver and decreased protein synthesis.

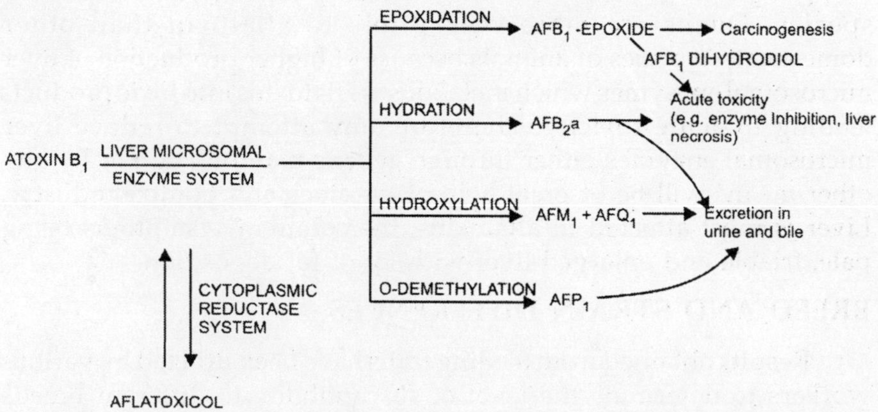

The adverse effects of aflatoxins in animals are characterized by lack of appetite, stunted growth, decreased egg production and egg weight and reproductive disorder in layers; decreased milk production and reproductive performance in dairy cattle; suppression of immune system leading to susceptibility to diseases, increased leg problems and decreased nutrient utilization. In case of severe aflatoxins, the net effect is usually grave.

GENETIC DIFFERENCES

Differences among individuals for susceptibility to the aflatoxins is well documented in literature. This may be either due to genetic or environmental factors or both. The susceptibility to aflatoxins is also influenced by other factors like energy intake management conditions, disease prevalence, general environmental and physiological stress, sex differences and nutritional status. The aflatoxins interact with DNA, depress the formation of messenger RNA and result in the decreased protein synthesis.

SPECIES DIFFERENCES

Differences among the species for susceptibility to aflatoxins was reported by Gumbmann *et al.* (1970), Muller *et al.* (1970). Cowell *et al.* (1973), Arafa and Blamer (1981) from feeding trials as well as from *vitro* studies. Among the domestic animals, ducks are more susceptible to aflatoxins followed by turkey poults, rabbits, dogs, pigs, calves, chickens, quails and sheep. Gossling and pheasants are more sensitive than chickens but definitely less sensitive than ducklings and turkey poults. Japanese quails and Bob White quails are also relatively more sensitive than chicken. From the available evidence, it appears that guinea fowls are less susceptible among the poultry species. Ducks are more susceptible to aflatoxin than other domesticated species of animals because of higher production of liver microsomal enzsymes which metabolises aflatoxins into toxic products leading to acute toxicity. Therefore, any attempt to reduce liver microsomal enzymes either through genetic manipulation or by any other means will be of great help of livestock and poultry industry. Liver is most affected in aflatoxins, the common sysmptoms being pale, friable and enlarged liver with lot of fat deposition.

BREED AND STRAIN DIFFERENCES

Results obtained from feeding trails have been utilized by various workers to determine the level of susceptibility to different breeds and strains of different breeds and strains of chickens to aflatoxins. These include the studies of Brown and Abram (1965), Carnaghan *et al.* (1967), Brown and Abram (*loc cit*) reported greater susceptibility for Newhamshire chicks than Cornish and Rhode Island Red chicks. Confirmatory results to this observation was reported by Florentine *et al.* (1969) through comparison of dietary aflatoxins in 10 different genetic groups such as Brahmas, Langshans, Rhode Island Reds, New Hampshire, Barred Plymouth Rocks and Single Comb White Leghorns and certain crossbred groups. Rate of growth and overall mortality to different diseases was used to measure the susceptibility to aflatoxins in this study. The results suggested that Brahmas was the most susceptible and White Plymouth the duck the least. Other confirmation to these results were also provided by Carnaghan *et al.* (1967) and Gumbmann (1970). In their study, Newhampshire chicks were found to be more susceptible and White Plymouth Rocks least susceptible. Leghorns and Rhode Island Reds were intermediate to these two extreme groups. Growth retardation was observed at feed levels of 500 ppb of aflatoxin in this study. The hybrid chicks, however, performed satisfactorily at somewhat higher levels of aflatoxins as there was little decline on their growth rate or egg yield.

Differences among the strains for susceptibility to aflatoxin was provided by Smith and Hamilton (1970). In comparison of the White Leghorn strains for body weight at six weeks of age, Smith and Hamilton observed considerable differences among the LD_{50} doses of aflatoxins. The differences between the most resistant and most susceptible strain was to the order of 2½ fold.

Williams *et al.* (1980) reported differences to aflatoxins sensitivity among 17 primary breeder strains using tracheal organ culture technique. Differences were also reported among the individuals of a strain in this study to aflatoxin AFB_1.

SEX AND AGE DIFFERENCES

The males are more sensitive to aflatoxins than females in Poultry (Brown and Abram, 1965); Carnaghan *et al.* (1970). Williams *et al.* (1980) Sub served sex related in *vitro* sensitivity to aflatoxin in two out of the three strains examined. According to Sharlin *et al.* (1980), the sex differences in sensitivity to aflatoxin may be attributed to the interaction of sex hormones with aflatoxin metabolism.

Asphin and Carnaghan (1961) and Brown and Abram (1965) reported greater susceptibility for young chick birds than adults. According to Smith and Hamilton (1970), the higher sensitivity of young birds are apparent only when susceptibility is measured in terms of growth rate as these differences were not well marked when defined in terms of actual LD_{50} values. In his study, older broilers appeared to be as susceptible as broilers ready for sale.

RESULTS FOR SELECTION

The differences among individuals, among the strains, among the breeds and among species suggest that susceptibility to aflatoxins in genetically inherited. With this inview, selection studies were undertaken by several workers to produce high susceptible and resistant strains of chickens to aflatoxins. Carnaghan *et al.* (1957) and Gumbmann *et al.* (1970) suggested a simple Mendelian inheritance for susceptibility to aflatoxins in chickens. According to them susceptibility is recessive to resistance and it is determined by single pair of autosomal genes.

Using family selection as criterion of selection, Marks and Wyatt (1979) developed less and more susceptible lines of quails by challenging them with 2.5 and 3.0 mg of aflatoxin per kg body weight. Selection through five generations showed rapid and continued reduction in mortality. Compared to control, there were 8 and 11 fold differences in the selected lines for mortality. This rapid initial response to selection and also results obtained from reciprocal crossing between the selected lines and base population showed than a few loci may be involved in determining resistance or susceptibility to aflatoxins to quail.

Williams *et al.* (1980) reported differences among individuals for susceptibility to aflatoxins. This study suggests that progeny testing may be suitable utilized for development of resistant strains for aflatoxins in poultry.

CONCLUSION

Some information, as available in literature on genetics of aflatoxicosis in avian species have been presented above. From this it would appear that genetic approach to aflatoxicosis may be a useful method compared to other methods for control of aflatoxocosis. It should, however, be remembered that resistance or susceptibility to aflatoxicosis is relative and not absolute like that of genetic resistance to disease. Further, I will like to say that we have no exact idea whether a few or more loci are involved in inheritance of susceptibility to aflatoxicosis. In view of the above, it appears that the solution for preventing aflatoxicosis in avian species is far from reality at present through utilization of genetical mechanisms.

REFERENCES

Arafa, A.S. and Blumer, R.J. 1931. Susceptibility of various poultry species of dietary aflatoxin. Br. Poult. Sci. 22: 431-436.

Asplin, F.D. and Carnaghan, R.B.A. 1961. The toxicity of certain ground nut meals for poultry with special reference to their effect on ducklings and chicken. Vet. Rec. 73: 1215-1218.

Brown. J.M.M. and Abrams, L. 1965. Biochemical studies on aflatoxicosis. Onderstepoort, J. Vet. Res. 32 119-172.

Colwell, W.M., Ashley, R.C., Simmons, D.G. and Hamilton, P.B. 1973. The relative invitro sensitivity to aflatoxin B1 of tracheal organ culture prepared from day-old chickens, ducks, Japanese quails and turkeys. Avian Dis. 17: 166-172.

Carnaghan, R.S.A., Nancy Hevert, C., Patterson, D.S.P. and Sweasey. D. 1987. Comparative biological and biochemical study in hybrid chicks, 2. Susceptibility to aflatoxin and effects on serum protein constituents. Brit. Poult. Sci., 8: 279-234.

Florentin, E.R., Cottier, G.L., Diener, U.L. and Davis, N.D. 1969. The effect of aflatoxin of different breeds and crosses of chickens. Poult. Sci. 48: 1307(Abstr).

Gumbmann, M.R., Williams, S.N., Booth, A.N., Vohra, P., Ernest, R.A. and Bethard, M. 1970. Aflatoxicosis in various breeds of poultry. Proc. Soc. Exptl. Biol. Med. 134: 683-688.

Marks, H.L. and Wyatt, R.D. 1970. Genetic resistance to aflatoxin in Japanese quails, Science, 206: 1329-1330

Smith, J.M. and Hamilton, P.B. 1970. Aflatoxicosis in the broiler chicken. Poult. Sci., 49: 207-215

Williams, C.M. Colwll, W.M. and Rose, L.P. 1980. Genetic resistance of chickens to aflatoxins assessed with organ culture techniques. Avian Dis. 24: 415-422.

Sharlin, J.S., Howarth, B. and Wyatt, R.D. 1980. Effect of dietary aflatoxin on reproductive performance of mature White Leghorn males. Poult. Sci., 59: 1311-1315.

CHAPTER

6

TRICHOTHECENES AND POULTRY DISEASES

S.M. Reddy

Department of Botany , Kakatiya University, Warangal 506 009.

INTRODUCTION

Trichothecenes are a group of fungal metabolites characterised by the *tetracyclic sesqueterpene 12, 13-epoxy-9-trichothecene* skeleton. The history of trichothecene mycotoxins goes back to the report of a trichothecene isolated as an antibiotic from *Trichotheceium roseum* by Freeman and Morrison (1949). However, the structure of these compounds have been elucidated by Godfredson *at at.* (1967). Another trichothecene called trichodermin was isolated as an antifungal metabolite of *Trichoderma viride.* Subsequently several trichothecenes were added to this list.

There are over 45-naturally occurring derivatives produced by different species of *Cephalosporium, Cylindrocarpon, Fusarium, Myrothecium, Stachybotrvs, Trichoderma, Trichothecium* and *Verticimonosporium* which are generally associated with the toxicity of mouldy cereal grains. Recently the structural elucidation of triepoxide trichothecene, baccharin, has been reported from a Brazilian plant (*Beccharis megapotanica*) (Kupchan, 1976).

The cultural conditions for production of different trichothecene differ widely. For production of antifungal trichothecenes such as trichothecin, trichodermin and crotocin, submerged culture is congenial. Surface culture is usually employed for trichothecenes such *as T-2* toxin. Neosolaniol is produced either in shake culture or by jar fermentation. The trichothecene compounds are usually colourless crystalline compounds. The biological activity of these compounds are attributed to the 12, 13-epoxytrichothecens. The structural alterations results in the modification of biological response (Ueno, 1977). The other common structural features of these compounds is 9, 10 double bond. The reduction of these bonds to give the corresponding dihydroderivitive consistently lead to the diminished cytotoxicity (Grave and Mortimer, 1969). Acetylation of some, but not all of the hydroxy substituents generally lead to the increased toxicity (Ueno, 1977). Introduction of hydroxyl group at appropriate position on the trichothecene skeleton often served to increase the biological activity.

Classification of trichothecenes

Trichothecene mycotoxins are mainly classified into five groups on the basis of chemical structures (Ueno, 1977).

Type A : hydroxyl-or acel-substituted trichothecene

Trichodermol
Trichodermin
Verrucarol
Scirpentriol
Monoacetoxy scrirpentriol
Diacetoxyscirpenol
7 , 8-Dihydroxydiacetoxyscirpeno
T-2 tetrol
T-2 toxin
T-2- toxin

Type B : 8 - Keto trichothecene

Trichothecolone
Trichothecin
Nivalenol
Fusarinone-X
Diacetylnivalenol
Deoxynivalenol
Tera acetylnivalinol

Type C : 7, 8 -Epoxy trichothecene

Crotocol
Crotocin

Type D : Verrucarins & Roridins

Verrucarin A
Verrucarin B
Verrucarin J
Roridin A

Roridin B

Type E : 7, 8-Epxoxy roridins

Epoxyisororidins E

Epoxyroridin H

Diepoxyroridin

The last two groups (4 & 5) are characterised by a macrocyclic ester or later-ether bridge between position C-4 and C-15 while the former three are non-microcyclic trichothecenes.

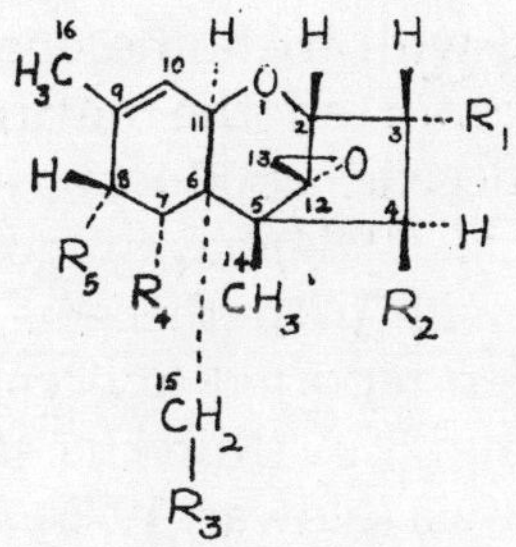

HYDROXYL OR ACYL-SUBSTITUTED TRICHOTHECENES

Among them A & B trichothecenes are important in practical analysis. Type A trichothecens are characterised by the hydrogen atom or a hydroxyl group on the 8 position in the trichothecene nucleus and type B by a carbonyl group.

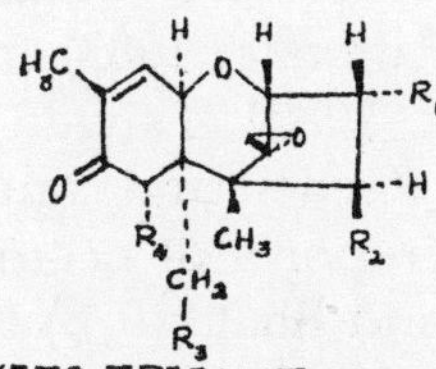

8-KETO TRICHOTHECENES

The multiplicity of trichothecene mycotoxins has been attributed to the ability of trichothecene producing *Fusarium* strains to acetylate or deacetylate exogenously supplied toxins, particularly deoxynivalenol, t-2 toxin and their derivatives (Yosizawa and Moroka, 1975a and b). Similarly Claridge and Schmidtz (1978) have reported that diacetoxyscirpenol could also be selectively deacetylated by cultures of *Streptomyces greseus* and *Acetanobacter calcoacetius* and acetylated by the fungus *Mucor mucedo.*

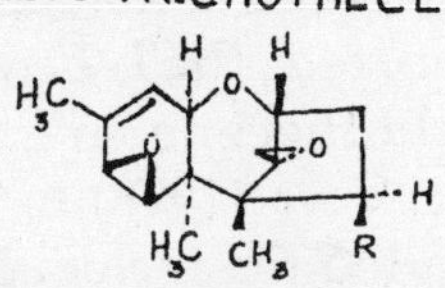

7-8 - EPOXYTRICHOTHECENES

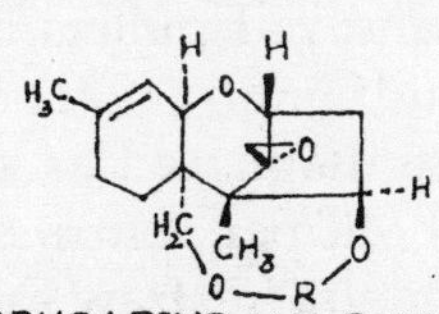

VERRUCARINS AND RORIDINS

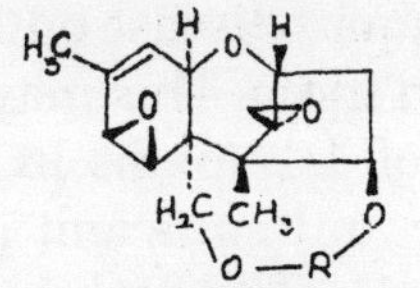

7,8 - EPOXYRORIDINS

Natural incidence

Natural occurrence of trichothecenes are high incidence of

fungi producing these toxins and production of these substances in various agricultural commodities such as cereals. Hsu *et al.* (1972) have reported the natural occurrence of trichothecenes in cattle feed and corn samples. Greenway and Puls (1976) and Mirocha *et al.* (1976b) have also reported the presence of *trichothecens* in barley and maize cereals. *Commercial pellets and mixed* feed in British Colombia Canada and US. Yoshizawa and Morcoka (1977) and Vesonder *et al.* (1978) have demonstrated heavy contamination of corn and barley in Japan and US with trichothecenes. Jemmali *et al.* (1978) and Szigeti (1976) have reported the natural contamination of barley seeds by trichothecene- producing fungi from France and Hungary. Recently Scott *et al.* (1984) have reported the contamination of wheat and other grains with trichothecene- producing fungi in Canada. These have also been reported to occur naturally from other parts of the world including USA (Mirocha *et al.* 1977 and Pathre and Mirocha, 1979), Yugoslavia (Nowar, 1975), North America (Vesonder, 1983), Portugal (cimeno, 1983), Canada (Scott *et al.* 1981 and Scott 1983), Japan (Kamimura *et al.* 1981 and Yoshizawa, 1983), Finland (Hintikka, 1983), Denmark (Pale and Bendicte, 1983), Britain (Patterson and Roberts, 1979 and Patterson, 1983), Italy (Giovanni, 1983), South Africa (Marasas and Krick, 1983), Taiwan (Tseng, 1983), France (Jamoa 1983) and Germany (Gedek and Bauer, 1983), However, there are only a few scattered reports of occurrance of trichothecene toxins in Indian Rukmini and Bhat (1978) have reported the occurrence of T-2 toxins in sorghum grains contaminated with head moulds. Ghosal *et al.* (1977) have reported theT-2 toxin, diacetoxyscirpenol and 12, 13-epoxytrichothecene in safflower seeds infected with *Fusarium oxysporum.* Vora (1978) in his survey of different parts of northern India reported the incidence of various species of *Fusarium.* Tripathi *et al.* (1968) have reported the death of 22 birds out of a flock of 236 Rhode Island red pullets in the Orissa state poultry breeding farm. Sharma and Singh (1971) and Rajendran *et al.* (1975) have reported the disease diagnosed as stachybotryotoxicosis, which involved 160 cattle with 40 per cent mortality was attributed to the presence of *Stachybotrysatra* in straw samples.

No human disease outbreak attribute to *Fusarium* toxins has been observed in India. This may not be entirely due to the absence or low incidence of T-2 toxins in Indian foods but may be due to lack of knowledge and sufficient information on epidemological aspects of mycotoxicosis. The high incidence of esophagus cancer in Transkei,

South Africa has been attributed to the high level of deoxynivalenol and zearalenone (Marasas *et al.*,1979).

Isolation and Detection method

Methods for this detection and analysis of the trichothecenes can be divided into two categories; 1. Physicochemical 2. Biological. Biological tests was highly sensitive but lack specificity, while physicochemical methods are generally specific. Foods and feeds are contaminated with variety of mycotoxins. Hence, simultaneous analysis by this layer chromatography is suitable for analysis of mycotoxins. The compounds detected either with UV, iodine vapour or by spraying the plate with different reagents such as Sulphuric acid (Gimeno, 1969), p-asnisaldehyde (Stahr *et al.*1979), aluminium chloride (Naoi *et al.*, 1974), 4-(paranitrobenyl) pyridine (Takitani *et al.* 1979) nicotinamide-2-acetylpyridine (Sano *et al.*1982) and Erlich reagent (Dowkins, 1966) are being used for the detection of trichothecene toxins on TLC plates.

Kamimura *et al.* have (1981) developed simultaneous detection of the trichothecene compounds. This is most simple, low cost and fact-detecting methods. The extract is applied on TLC plates and run in different solvents. The compounds are detected by using different spraying reagents.

A lack of spetral and chemical properties which permit the detection of trichothecenes in small quanities, a gas liquid chromatography assay was developed. Pryex columns were used regularly in the gas-liquid chromatographic studies. Kamimura (1981) reported a method for concomitant analysis of trichothecenes.

These toxins can also be detected by various biological tests. Muller and Lepom (1985) have recommended the use of larvae of *Artemia salina* as a bioassy agent for the detection of trichothecene toxin in maize. Gilgan *et al.* (1966) and Bamburg, (1968) have introduced the skin toxicity test for the detection of toxigenic *Fusarium* species and their metabolites from mouldy corn. Chung *et al.* (1974) have proposed rabbit bioassay test for large number of field samples of corn for trichothecene toxins.

Biological activity

a) Animal disease:

Vomiting and feed refusal are common toxicological features of trichothecene type of mycotoxins. Staggering toxicoses Siberia, Elementary toxic alekia in Russia, red mould disease in Japan mouldy corn toxicoses in United States, Stachybotriotoxicosis in Hungary, dendrotoxicosis in Central Europe and related toxicoses have been reported to be characteristic symptoms of trichothecene compounds.

The trichothecene compounds have been reported to possess a potent cytotoxicity to eukaryotes (Chtsubo and Saito, 1970). Eppley (1974) developed a bioassay method for the detection of trichothecene using brino shrimp larvae (*Artemia salina L.*). Several approaches have been made to demonstrate the phytotoxicity of trichothecenes. A quantitative bioassay method using pea seeds has been developed by Marasas *et al.* (1971). Pollen germination of *Nicotiana sylvestris* has also been used as a bioassay agent. The well known and best bioassay method is antimicrobial activity. Biochemical assay method was reported by Foster *et al.* (1975). The 12, 13-epoxy trichothecenes react with glutathinae and glutathiane epoxide transferease catalyzes this conjugation reaction. Recently, radioimmuno assay and enzyme-linked immunosorbank assay have been developed for detection of these mycotoxins. (Chu *et al.*, 1979).

Toxicity of trichothecenes is highest in type C compounds such as verrucarin A and roridin A, followed by type A, e.g. T-2 toxin and type B, e.g. nivalenol. Nonmacrocyclic compounds of crotocin (type D) is the least toxic trichothecene.

Pharmacological investigations with fusaranon-X revealed that this mycotoxin induced hypothermia (Matauoka*et al.*, 1979). Diarrhea is one of the characteristic response of animals administered with a sublethal dose of toxins (Matsuoka and Kubota, 1982).

b) Poultry Disease:

I Chi *et al.* (1977) have observed the following symptoms of T-2 toxins.

1. Decrease in feed consumption
2. Decrease in egg production
3. Decrease in thickness of egg shell
4. Hatchability is affected adversely
5. Uric acid accumulation
6. Prusa of faricius was reduced in weight
7. Increasing weight of liver, pancreas

Wyett *et al.* (1973) have observed following the symptoms in toxin and fed chicks

II.1. Decrease in growth gain

2. Inflamatory, necrotic intestinal lesions
3. Haemorrhage in heart muscles and liver muscles
4. Affect of lipid metabolism cause decrease in vitamin E
5. Neural disturbances

Yoshizawa (1980) feels that T_2-toxin is metabolized into more toxin polor derivatives and excretion in the urine. Deacetion and hydroxylation results in subsequent decreased toxicity of T_2-toxin.

III Effect of Zearalenone on chicks

1. Drop in egg
2. Egg size decreased
3. Hyperesterogenic response
4. Enlargement of cloacal bursa
5. Oviduct enlargement

C. General toxic symptoms of trichothecenes produced by Fusarium Spp.

The characteristic of the first stage include primary changes in the buccal cavity and gastriointestinal tract, the patients feels a burning sensation in the mouth, tongue, throat, palate, esophague and stomach as the toxin acts on the mucosa of the oral cavity may be hypermic. Inflamation of the gastric and intestinal mucosa result in vomiting, diarrhoea and abdominal pain.

The leucocyte count may decrease in first stage of level 2000 min^3 and there may be increased erythrocyte sedimentation rate (Yefremov, 1948).

Latent stage is called second stage and also called the leuekopenic stage. the patient feels well and is capable of normal activity (Romonova, 1947) normal duration of the stage is usually from 3-4 weeks.

1. Progressive leukopenia
2. Granulopenia
3. Relative hymphocytosis
4. Anemia

5. Decrease in number of eucocytes
6. Changes in the resistance of the body to bacterial infection.
7. Changes in hepatopoietic system
8. Disturbance of central and autonomic nervous system
9. Weakness, headache
10. Mils asthamatic cystonus.
11. There may be diarrhoea.

If the consumption of the toxic grain continues, the symptoms of the third stage rapidly developed.

Transition stage is sudden from second stage. The first visible sign of the third stage is hemorrhage on the skin of trunk, in the axillary and on the lateral surface of the arms and thigh and serious cases on the face and head.

1. Haemorrhage may be found on mucous membranes, mouth, tongue, nasal, gastric and intestinal.
2. Necrotic changes soon appears in the throat, changes may extend to the buccal mucosa, vocal chord, lips, skin of the nose, jaws, and eyes.
3. Usually contaminated with different variety of avirulent bacteria.
4. Unpleasant odour from the mouth due to the bacteria infection because of enzymatic activity of bacteria on proteins.
5. The lymphocytes may constitues 90% of the white cells present, blood sedimentation rate in increased.

Fourth stage:

This is a stage of convolescence and depend on the intensity of the toxicoses.

REFERENCES

Bamburg, J.R., N.V. Riggs and F.M. Strong, *Tetrahydron Lett. 24,* 1968, 3329.

Chu, F.S., S. Grossman, R.D. Weiand, C.J. Mirocha, *Appl. Environ. Microbiol,* 1979, 104.

Chung, C.W., M.W.Truckness, A.L. Giles, Jr. and L. Friedman, *J. Assoc. Off. Anal. Chem., 54,* 1874, 1121.

Chi, M.S., C.J. Mirocha, H.J. Kurtz, G. Weaver, F. Bates, W. Shinoda, *Poultry Sci., 56,* 1977, 628.

Claridge, C.A. and H. Schmitz, *Appl, Environ. Microbiol. 36.* 1978, 63.

Dowkins, A.W., *J. Chem. Soc., 116,* 1966.

Eppley, R.M., *J. Assoc, Off. Anal. Chem., 57,* 1974, 618.

Foster, P.M., T.F., Shater and D.S.P. Pattersan, *Biochem. Soc. Trans., 3,* 1975, 875.

Freaman, G.G. and R.I. Morrison, *Biochem, J., 44.* 1949, 1.

Gedeck. B. and J. Bauer, Trichothecenes, Chemical, Biological, and Toxicological Aspects, (ed. Y. Ueno) Elsevir Publi, 1983, 301.

Ghosal, S., D.K. Chakrabarti and K.C. Chautary, *Experientia. 33,* 1977, 574.

Gilgan, M.W., E.B. Smalley and F.M. Strong, *Arch Biochem, Biophys. 114,* 1966, 1.

Gimeno, A., *J. Assoc. Off. Anal. Chem. 62,* 1979, 579.

Gimeno, A., *J. Assoc. Off. Anal. Chem. 66,* 1983, 565.

Giovanni, C., Trichothecene-Chemical, Biological and Toxicological Aspects, (Ed. Y. Ueno), Elasevir Publish, 1983, 254.

Godt Fredson, W.O., J.F. Grove and Ch. Tamm, *Helv. Chim. Acta- 50.* 1967. 1666.

Greenway, J.A. and R. Puls, *Can . J.Camp. Med. 40.* 1976, 12.

Grove, J.F. and P.H. Mortimer, *Biochem. Pharmacol. 18,* 1969, 1473.

Kamimura, H., M. Nishijama, K. Yasuda, K. Saito, A. Ibe, T. Nagayam,a H. Usliyama and Y. Naoi, *J. Assooc. Off. Chem. 64,* 1981, 1067.

Hsu, I.C., E.B., Smalley, F.M. Strong and W.E. Ribilin, *Appl. Microbiol. 24,* 1972, 684.

Jemeli, M., Trichothecenes-Chemical, Biological and Toxicological Aspects (ed. Y. Ueno), Elsvir Publish 1983, 297.

Jemeli, M., Y. Ueno, K. Ishil, C. Frassinet and M. Ethinne, *Experientia, 34,* 1978, 1333.

Kaminura, H., *Proc, Jap. Assoc, Mycotoxical, 43,* 1981.

Kupchan, S.M., B.B. Jarvis, R.G., Bailey Jr., W. Bright, R.F. Byran and Y. Shizuri, *Food Cosmet. Toxicol. 10,* 1976, 501.

Marasas, W.F.O., E.B., Smalley, J.R., Banburg and F.M. Strong. *Phytopathology, 61,* 1971, 1488.

Marasas, W.F.O. and N.P.J. Krick, Trichothecene—Chemical, Biological and Toxicological Aspects (ed. Y. Ueno), Elasver Publi, 1983, 273.

Marsas, W.F.O., S.J. Van Rensburg and C.J. Mirocha, *Ja. Agric, Food, Chem.*

Matasuka Y., and K. Kuboto, *J. Pharm. Dym. 5,* 1982, 193.

Matasuka, Y., and K. Kuboto and Y. Ueno, *Toxicol. Appl. Pharmacol. 50,* 1979, 87.

Mirocha, C.J. S.U. Pathre, B. Schauerhamer and C.M. christensen, *Appl. Environm. Microbiol. 32,* 1976, 553.

Mirocha, C.J., S.U. Pathre, and C.M. Christensen, Mycotoxin fungi Mycotoxins, Microtoxicosis, *1*, Marcel Dekker, Inc., New York 1977, 365.

Naoi. Y., e. Kazana, K. Saito, H. Ogawa, K. Shimura and Y. Kimura, *Ann, Rept. Tokyo, Ketr, Res. Lab. P.H. 25*, 1974, 203.

Nowar, M.E., Ph. D. thesis, Navisad University, Yugoslavia, 1975.

Ontsubo, K. and M. Saiton *Japan J. Exp. Med. 23*, 1970, 217.

Palle, K. and H. Bendicte, Trichothecenes-chemical, Biological and Toxicological Aspects, (ed. Y. Ueno). Elasvir Publi 1983, 151.

Pathre, S.V. and C. J. Mirocha, *J. Amer. Oil Chem. Soc. 56*, 1979, 820.

Patterson, D.S.P. and B.A. Roberts, *J. Assoc. Anal. Chem. 62*, 1979, 1265.

Patterson. D.S.P. Trichothecens Chemical, Biological and Toxicological Aspects, (ed. Y. Ueno), Elsvir Publi, 1983, 259.

Rajendran, M.P., M.J. Hussain and K. Ramni, *Inidan, Vet. J. 52*, 1975, 234.

Rukinimi, C. and R.V. Bhat, *J. Agri, Food Chem. 26*, 1978, 647.

Sano, A., Y. Asabe, S. Takitani and Y. Ueno, *Ja. chromatogr. 235*, 1982, 257.

Scott, D.M., Trichothecenes, Chemical, Biological and Toxicological Aspects, (ed. Ueno), Elsvir Publi, 1983, 218.

Szigeti, G, Ph.D. Thesis, Miskok, Hungary, 1976.

Sharma, U.K. and N. Singh, *Indian, Vet J. 44*, 1971.

Stahr, H.M., A. A. Karaft and M. Schuh, *Appl. spectosc. 33*, 1979, 294.

Scott, P.M., P.Y. Lau and S.R. Kanhere, *J. Assoc. Off. Anal. Chem.64*, 1981, 1364.

Takitani, S., Y. Asabe, T. Kalo, M. Suzuki and Y. Ueno. *J. Charamotogr.172*, 1979, 335.

Tripatty, S.B., N.C., Nayak and K.M. Mohanty. *Indian Vet J. 44*, 1967, 813.

Tseng, T. Trichothecene-Chemical, Biological and Toxicological Aspects (ed. Y. Ueno). Elsvir Publi. 1983, 290.

Ueno, Y., *Pure Appl, Chem. 49*, 1977, 1737.

Ueno, Y. Mycotoxin in Human and Animal Health (ed. J.V. Rodricks, C.W. Hessel tine and M.A. Machiman), 1977, 193, Pathotax Publishers.

Vesonder, R.F. Trichothecenes-Chemical, Biological and Toxicological Aspects (ed. Y. Ueno), Elsevier Publi., 1983, 210.

Vesonder, R.F., A. Ciegler, R.F. Rogers, K.A. Burbridge, R.J. Bothert, and A.H. Jensen. *Appl. Environ, Microbiol. 36*, 1978, 885.

Vora, V.C. *Central Drug Research Institute* Lucknow, 1978, 13.

Wyatt, R.D., P.B. Hamilton and H.R. Burmeister, *Poultry Sci. 52*, 1973, 1853.

Yefremov, U.V. *Publ. Med. Ltd. Moscow.* 1948, 118.

Yoshizawa, T., Trichothecenes-Chemical, Biological and Toxicological Aspects (ed. Y. Ueno), Elsevir Publ. 1983, 195.

Yoshizawa, T. and N. Morooka, *Appl. Microbiol. 29,* 1975a, 54.

Yoshizawa, T. and N. Morooka, *Appl. Microbiol.30,* 1975b, 38.

Yoshizawa, T. and N. Morooka, Mycotoxins in Human and Animal Health (J.V. Rodricks, C.W. Hesseltine and M.A. Mehlman, eds) Pathotox, 1977, 309.

Yoshizawa, T., S. Swanson and C.J. Mirocha, *Appl. Environ. Microbiol. 40,* 1980, 901.

CHAPTER

7

PATHOLOGY OF FOOD-BORNE MYCOTOXIN IN POULTRY

Dr. S.M. Mohiuddin
Associate Professor & Head, Department of Pathology, Veterinary College, Rajendranagar, Hyderabad.

INTRODUCTION

Mycotoxins, a group of metabolites elaborate by fungi, in the media in which they grow are of great significance in the health of man and livestock then we realize. Although as many as 100 species of fungi are common in feeds, only few fungi which are responsible to produce potent toxins have been identified. The prominence of mycotoxins in livestock production was realized only after Turkey X disease involving the death of large number of turkeys during 1960 in England.

Health hazards have become a major problem of poultry industry in spite of various prophylactic and therapeutic methods used for various disease. Mycotoxicosis is one of the major causes of many unknown disease problems, which cause economic losses to poultry by affecting body weight gain, low egg production and mortality of birds. Besides this, it is also important from the public health point of view since these toxins and their metabolites are present in poultry products which are harmful to human beings also.

In this paper, an attempt has been made to discuss the various effects of Aflatoxins, produced to *Aspergillus flavus;* Ochratoxin produced by *Aspergillus ochaceus* : Zeralenone produced by *Fusarium germination,* Citrium produced by *P. citricum* : Sterigmatocystin produced by *Aspergillus versicolour* and T.2 toxin produced by *F. trichintum., F. roseum* and *F. oxysporum.*

A. Aflatoxins

Aspergillus flavus and Aspergillus parasiticus are the two most important species which produce aflatoxins. The aflatoxins are a mixture of toxin metabolites i.e. B_1, B_2, G_1, G_2, M_1 and M_2 with B_1 as most potent and toxic product. Aflatoxins are extremely hepatotixic, mytagenic and carcinogenic to livestock and poultry. The order of susceptibility among poultry is in ducklings which are highly susceptible followed by turkey poults, gooslings, chicken and quails.

Pathology

In Aflatoxicosis the growth rate isdecreased as a result of altered protein metabolism and hence affected birds have poor feed conversion. This brings about its toxic effect by interfering fat transport in the liver and thus cause the liver to become pale and large. In layers, there is a drop in productionand decreases hatchability without affecting the fertility. In broiler chicken, aflatoxin causes decreased growth and feed conversion. In acute toxicity mortality is high with enlarged liver and spleen ; regressed bursa of fabricius, pale comb, shank and bone marrow. In general aflatoxin in poultry can cause haemorrhagic anemia syndrome characterised by petechial and larger haemorrhages.

The susceptibility to aflatoxin vary markedly in different avian species. the young in all species were more susceptible than adults. Ducklings and turkey poults were more susceptible than most breeds of poultry. In ducklings aflatoxin causes convulsion and purple discoloration of shanks and web associated with severe lameness. Affected birds die within a week and assume a characteristic posture, the head is drawn back and legs extended fully backwards. The lesions include enlargement of liver, with haemorrhages and at time necrotic lesions. The kidneys are usually swollen.

Histopathogically, the liver cells showed degenerative changes, viz., cloudy swelling to fatty changes depending upon the acute nature of the condition. These changes are periportal in distribution. There will be extensive proliferation of bile epithelum. At times nodular or discrete hyperplasia of the portal spaceses, occlusion of hepatic sinusoides and enlargement of hepatic nuclei will be noticed. In kidneys glomerular hyperplasia discrete glomerulosclerosis vascular degeneration of tubules will be noticed.

Asplin and Carnaghan (1961) and Carnaghan *et al.* (1966) observed enlarged and grey-coloured livers in chickens receiving experimental diets containing 1.5 ppm of aflatoxin. The consistency of the liver was soft with petechial haemorrhages. Thereafter there was a reduction in size of the liver with increasing firmness and texture until the 7th week, with well-defined, raised nodular lesions on the liver surface, diffuse white pinhead sized foci were found from the sixth week of age.

Archibald *et al.* (1962) noticed pale enlarged kidneys and had a fine network of urate deposite. While Newberne (1965) reported swollen and pale brown kidneys, protein debris was present in abnormal quantities in dilated tubules with a large nuclei of the degenerating epithelial cells.

Birds receiving diet containing 0.5, 1.0 ppm aflatoxin reported to have shown no gross lesions, while at 2.0 ppm to 4 ppm levels livers appeared pale and lighter compared to normal (Muller *et al.*,1970).

Vanzytveld *et al.* (1970) have observed in the dead broiler chicks administered with 256.6 ug to 513.0 ug of aflatoxin, into crop daily for 6 weeks mottled appearance and of liver and small reddish spots of 1 to 2 mm size, which tended to be firm, and the edges somewhat rounded. No evidence of nodule formation was observed. Liver colour varied from slightly pale to intense pale yellow kidneys and spleen were usually pale in affected birds.

Yadgiri (1970) observed, diffuse liver cell necrosis, shrunken cells withbpyknotic nuclei, fatty vacuolation in the cytoplasm, of liver cells in ducks. The liver cell damage has always been more severe in the periportal zones than in the centrilobular zones and mild bile duct proliferation.

Aflatoxin in the diet increased the weight of liver and its content and the appearance of the liver was similar to that reported in fatty liver syndrome (Hamilton and Garlich, 1971). Tung *et al.* (1971) reported that small amounts of aflatoxin of the diet increased capillary fragility and susceptibility to bruising.

Dikman (1972) observed necrotic foci in spleen and heart apex. Granulamatous and tumoruous lesion in intestinal, epicardial, pericardial cutaneous, subcutaenous and muscular tissues head, leg and around hip joints in Aspergillus infection in broilers.

The bursa and thymus was atrophied at higher doses of aflatoxin. With inhibition of antibody formation (Thaxton *et al.* 1974).

Peckham (1975) reviewed the aflatoxin lesions in ducklings. They were hydropericardium, petichae on the pancreas, diffuse haemorrhages on kidney, enlarged gall bladder and duodenal inflammation.

Aflatoxin affects the cellular integrity of the host (Doerr *et al.* 1978) and also predisposes the birds to microbial and other diseases

(Wong and Hsieh, 1980).

Tapia *et al.* (1980) reported the presence of enlarged and pale liver, with severe degenerative lesions and proliferation of hepatocytes in the periportal region.

Mohiuddin (1982) reported that feeding of aflatoxin 100 and 200 ug/day/diet for 35 days resulted in atrophy of testes and absence of spermutogenesis, while the liver showed only congestion.

A Hypocarotenoidaemia and hepatic hyperlipaemia were seen during chronic aflatoxicosis in broiler chicks (Doerr *et al.*, 1983).

Moorthy *et al.* (1985) observed hepatic lesions in chickens given 6.25 ppm and 3.12 ppm aflatoxin in feed. Important gross lesions include pale yellow livers with haemorrhages, haematomas and nudules. The important histological findings were lipidosis, sinusoid congestion, perivascular haemorrhages, bileduct hyperplasia, phlebities and veno-occulusive lesions.

Mohiuddin *et al.* (1986) reported periportal fatty change, loss of normal hepatic architecture necrosis of hepatic cells with prominent kupffer in chicken fed aflatoxin 20 ppm for 3 months.

B. Ochratoxin

Ochratoxins are the most widely recognized toxin produced by *A. ochraceus,* a culture of *Aspergillus ochraceus.* The moulds producing the toxin was widely distributed in soil and decaying organic matter and frequently associated with mouldy feed.

Ochratoxin has been identified as Ochratoxin A, B and C, Ochratoxin A and C were toxin, while B was not toxic.

The LD_{50} of ochratoxin A for one day old ducklings is 25 ug and for chickens is 216 ug. Ochratoxin is the most toxin among all the metabolites.

Aspergillus ochraceus (Vander Merwe *et al.*, 1965a) produces ochratroxins, affect many animals and cause death in chickens also. In 14-week-old WLH chickens, ochratoxin causes retardation of sexual maturity and feeble egg production at low concentrations, and at higher concentrations, a very low egg production with hepatic and renal disorders. It reduces hatchability of fertile eggs and depressed subsequent performance of the progeny for their first two weeks of life. Suppression of haemopoiesis in the bone marrow and the depletion of lymphoid elements in the spleen and bursa of fabricus were predominent findings in chicks. Catarrhal entritis with heterophils in dilated intestinal glands, localised necrosis in renal tubules and urate deposition in ureters.

Theron *et al.*(1965) reported the ochratoxicosis in ducklings cause in increase in fatty vacuolation, changes in the matrix of the mitochondria, and disorganization of the endoplasmic reticulum of hepatocytes.

Doupnik and Peckham (1970) and Peckham *et al.* (1971) studied ochratoxicosis in young WLH cockerels, and reported postmortem dehydration emaciation, altered mucosal linings of gizzard, a few small haemorrhages in the proventriculus and enteritis while the main gross finding was visceral gout. Histopathologically there was actute nephrosis, hepatic degeneration and suppression of haematopoiesis.

Tucker and Hamilton (1971) reported that ochratoxin caused pathological changes in chickens such as emaciation, altered linings of the gizzard and increased liver glycogen.

Huff *et al.* (1974) studies ochratoxicosis of broiler chicken and noticed enlarged kidney, crop proventriculus, gizzard and liver, while the bursa of fabricium was regressed. Enlarged kidneys and reduced growth rates are most sensitive indicators. the pathological lesions include petichae on the papillae of proventriculus, slight gizzard erosions and paleness of the kidney, liver and pancreas.

Huff *et al.* (1975) reported enlarged kidneys, impaired renal function, increased uric acid production and concluded that ochratoxin is a severe nephrotoxin in young broiler chickens.

Chang *et al.* (1979) reported that ochratoxin -A induces a severe leucocytopenia (primarily) and monocytopenia to a lesser extent and implied that functioning of the immune system might be affected.

Ochratoxin-A induces impaired phagocytic ability of heterophils (Chang and Hamilton, 1980) and thymus regression in brolier chicken (Chang *et al.*, 1981)

Hamilton *et al.* (1982) observed an increased incidence of airsacculitis in severel field outbreak of ochratoxicosis in broiler fowls and related it to the possible immunosuppressive effects of the mycotoxin.

In young broiler chicks, ochratoxin A caused a significant enlargement of the kidney, liver and proventriculus, whereas the thymus and the bursa of fabricius were reduced in size. It principally affected the proximal convoluted tubules of the kidney causing severe distention, enlargement and hypertropy resulting in thickening of the glomercular basement membrane. In the liver vacuolation and glycogen accumulation in the hepatocytes, also regression of the lymphoid cell population in the immunological organs (Dwivedi and Burns, 1984).

Dwivedi *et al.* (1984) reported the following ultrastructural changes in the liver and kidneys in ochratoxicosis-A in the young broiler chicks. There was increased accumulation of cytoplasmic glycogen in the hepatocytes, abnormal mitochondrial ring formation in kidneys was reported in ochratoxicosis-A in young broiler chicks (Dwivedi, *et al.,* 1984 and Burns and Dwivedi, 1986).

Ochratoxin-A caused a significant depression in immunoglobulin containing cells in all the lymphoid organs studies (Dwivedi and Burns, 1984).

Bodnarchuk and Kaspruk (1984) reported the presence of haemorrhages in various tissues and catarrhal gastritis and enteritis.

Feeding ochratoxin-A from 0 to 21 days of age was associated with proximal tubular intranuclear membrane-bound inclusions, elongated tortuous and ring-shaped mitochondria, enlarged mitochondrial matrical granules with hyaline centres and an increase in size and membrane perisomes and secondary lyposomes (Brown *et al.,*1986).

C. Citrinin

Citrinin is an important toxin, production of which is mainly associated with *Pencillium citrium* and related species. This species has been frequently isolated from mouldy groundnuts. It forms grey green colonies which become grey, or olive green, as the spores mature, in the media.

Carlton (1980) noted that principal histological lesions in the kidney and the nephrotoxic effects of citrinin were considered the principal cause of death.

Citrinin is essentially toxic to kidneys and liver histopathological alterations in birds were most prominent in the kidneys which include degeneration and necrosis of tubular epithelial cells of both the proximal and distal convulted tubules. Hepatic lesions were multiple foci of necrosis. Haemorrhages, lymphoid necrosis and depletion were found in the bursa of fabricius, thymus, caecal tonsil and spleen in birds (Mehdi *et al.*, 1981)

Mehdi *et al.* (1984) observed that the mycotoxin was nephrotoxic and renal lesions were more severe in turkey than ducklings; and were characterized by degeneration and necrosis of renal tubular epithelium. Further hepatic cell necrosis and biliary hyperplasia were also noted in liver.

Hnatow and Wideman (1985) reported that citrinin acts directly on the kidneys to act several tubular transport process. These include increase in urinary flow rate, free water clearance and in sodium potassium and inorganic phosphate excretion.

Feeding citrinin from 1 to 21 days of age was associated with proximal tubular nuclear inclusions, elongated tortuous and ring-shaped mitochondria and an increase in size and number and peoxisomes and secondary lysosomes (Brown *et al.*, 1986).

D. Sterigmatocystin

Toxicosis which involve *A. versicolor* are probably due to sterigmatocystin, and related metabolites, which it produces. Sterigmatocystin itself is a pale yellow crystal line compound, which is insoluble in water.

Sterigmatocystin, at doses varying from 18-100 mg/kg causes liver necrosis which may be either centrilobular (when administered orally) or perioportal (when administered I/P). When the dose is very high (144 mg/kg) haemorrhages and severe necrosis of the tubules and glomerulus of the kidney are seen.

Sterigmatocystin is metabolized and secreted within 12-24 hrs in the urine, faeces and especially in the gastrointestinal tract of chicken.

Histopathological changes in the livers of ducklings fed sterigmatocystin produced by *A. versicolor* were, haemorrhages, hepatic parencghymal degeneration, necrosis, fatty changes, fibroblast proliferation and mitotic figures of the bile duct cells (Yoon, 1983).

Gross and histological examination revealed ruptured egg follicles swollen kidneys, which dilated tubules and haemorrhages, petechial haemorrhages in fatty tissues and degenerative changes in the nuclei of hepatocytes (Pojanvirta *et al.*, 1984).

Ivanokakii (1986) observed on postmortem hepatic degeneration, catarrhal enteritis and subcapsular haemorrhages in kidneys, at a dosage varying from 40-400 mg/kg BW.

E. Zearalenone

fusarium graminearum is the principle organism which produces Zearalenone. The mould is frequently seen on rye, oats, barley and rarely in rice. The infection of barley may be detected by a discolouration of the spikelet which becomes yellowish and then, brownish. Sometimes a red eflorescence of mycelium is visible on the surface.

The symptoms of toxicity include mainly disorders of the digestive tract accompanied by diarrhoea, often with blood faeces. There is weight loss, and a general loss of appetite. Frequent haemorrhagic lesions are also noted in the stomach, heart, intestines and lungs.

When turkey poults were fed a diet containing 300 ppm zearalenone or a diet composed of fusarium invaded corn at a level of 10#, swelling of the vent, mucous, secretion, and cystine, development in the cloaca occurred (Meronuck *et al.*, 1970).

Speers *et al.*, (1971) reported that the feeding of zearalenone or fusarium invaded corn (300 to 1600 ppm) to 10 days old WLH chicks did not cause any prominent signs except for an increase in weight gain and high incidence of cystine development in the genital tract.

F. T2 Toxin

It is produced by a variety of moulds viz., *F. fricinctum, F roseum* and *F. oxysporum.* The clinical signs are reduced feed intake and growth reduction ; reduced egg production and hatchability of fertile eggs and immuno-suppression. It is potent inhibitor of protein and DNA synthesis.

Mouth lesions are prominent. Caseous type of mouth lesions noticed in all parts of the mouth, reduction in feed intake, growth retardation, reduced hatchability and immunosuppression as they are potent inhibitors of protein and DNA synthesis.

REFERENCES

Archibald, R.M., H.J., Smith and J.D. Smith, 1962. Brazilian groundnut toxicosis in Canadian broiler chickens. Can. Vet. J. **3**(1) : 322-325.

Asplin, F.D. and B.A. Carnaghan. 1961. The toxicity of certain groundnut meals for poultry with special reference to their effect on ducklings are chickens. Vet. Rec. **73**(3) : 1215-1219.

Bodnarchuk, A.I. and I.M. Kaspruk. 1984. Ochratoxicosis in ducks. Poult. Abstr. **19**(5) : 1092 (Abstr.)

Brown, T.P., R.O. Manning, O.J. Fletcher and R.D. Wyatt. 1986. The individual and combined effects of citrinin and ochratoxin A on renal structure in layer chicks. Avian Diseases **30**(1) : 191-198.

Burns, R.B. and P.D. Dwivedi. 1986. The natural occurrence of ochratoxin A and its effects in poultry. A review. II. Pathology and immunology. World Poult. Sci. **42**(1) : 48-55.

Carlton, W.W. 1980. Citrine : In conference on mycotoxins in animal and feed and grains related to animal health pp. 275-323. Food and Drug Adm., US Dept. of Commerce, National Technical Information Service, USA.

Carnaghan, R.B.A., G. Lewis, D.S.P. Patterson and Ruth Allcroft. 1966. Biochemical and pathological aspects of groundnut poisoning in chickens. Pathol. Vet. 3 : 601-615.

Chang, C.F., J.A., Doerr and P.B. Hamilton, 1981. Comparative stud of T-2 toxin ochratoxin and aflatoxin in broiler chicken. Poult Sci. **60** (1) : 114-119.

Chang, C.F. and Hamilton. P.B. 1980. Ochratoxicosis in broiler chicken. Applied and Environment Microbiology. **39** (2) : 572-575.

Chang, C.F., W.E. Huff and P.B. Hamilton. 1979. A leucocytopenia induced in chickens by dietary ochratoxin. Poult. Sci., **58** (2) : 555-558.

Dijkman, K.E. 1972. Aspergillus flavus infections in broilers and its significance in poultry carcass infection. Tijdischrift voor Diergeness, Kunde, **97** : 1455.

Doerr, J.A., W.E. Huff and P.B. Hamilton. 1978. Enhanced susceptibility to bacterial toxins during aflatoxicosis. Poult. Sci. **57** (4) : 1134.

Doupnik B. and J.C. Peckham. 1970. Mycotoxicity of Aspergillus ochracens to chicks, Appl. Microbiol. **19** : 594-597.

Doerr, J.A., W.E. Huff and C.J., Wabeck, 1983. Effects of low level chronic aflatoxicosis in broiler chickens. Poult. Sci. **62** (10) : 1971-1977.

Dwivedi, P. and R. B. Burns, 1984. Pathology of ochratoxicosis A in young broiler chicks. Reseach Vet. Sci. **36** (1) : 92-103.

Dwivedi, P. and R.B. Burns, 1984. Effect of ochratoxin A on immunoglobulins in broiler chicks. Res. Vet. Sci. **36** (1) : 117-121.

Dwivedi, P., R. B. Burns and M. H. Maxwell. 1984. Ultrastructual study of the liver and kidney in ochratoxicosis A in young broiler chicks. res. Vety. Sci. **36** (1) : 104-116.

Hamilton. P.B., W.E. Huff, Haris, Jr., U.R.D. Wyatt. 1982. Pathology of ochratoxin in broiler fowls. Poult. Sci. **16** (4) : 1832-1841.

Hnatow, L.L. and R.F. Wideman, Jr. 1985. Kidney function of single comb white leghorn following acute renal portal poisoning of the mycotoxin Citrinin. Poult. Sci. 64(8) : 1553-1561.

Huff, W.E., R.D. Wyatt, T.L. Tucker and P.B. Hamilton. 1974. Ochratoxicosis in the broiler chickens. Poult. Sci. **53** (4) : 1585-1591.

Huff, W.E., R.D. Wyatt and P.B. Hamilton. 1975. Nephrotoxicity of dietary ochratoxin A in broiler chicken. Appl. Microbiol. **30** (1) : 48-51.

Ivanovskii, A.A. 1986. Effect of sterigmato cystin on fowls and on the quality of poultry meat. Poult. Abstr. **12** (2) : 3085 (Abstr).

Mehdi, N.A.Q., W.W. Carlton and J. Tuite. 1981. Citrinin mycotoxicosis in broiler chickens. Food and Cosmetics Toxicology **19**(6) : 723-733.

Mehdi, N.A.Q., W.W. Carlton and J. Tuite. 1983. Acute toxicity of citrinin in turkeys and ducklings. Avian Pathol. **12** (2) : 221-223.

Mehdi, N.A.Q, W.W. Carlton. G.D., Boon and J. Tuite, 1984. Studies on the sequential development and pathogenesis of citrinin mycotoxicosis in turkeys and ducklings, Vet. pathol. 21(2) : 216-223.

Mohiuddin, S.M. 1982. Note on the effect of aflatoxin on testis in poultry. Indian J. Anim. Sci. **52**(6) : 481-482.

Mohiuddin, S.M., M. Vikram Reddy, M. Madhya Reddy and K. Rama Krishan. Studies on phagocytic activity and haematological changes in aflatoxicosis in poultry. Indian Vet. J. **63** : 442-445.

Mornuck. R.A., K. H., Garren, C. M. Christensen. G. H. Nelson and F. Bates, 1970. Effects of turkey poults and chicks of rations containing corn invaded by pencillum and fusarium species. Amer. J. Vet. Res. **32** (2) : 551-556.

Moorthy, A.S., M. Mahender and P. R. Rao. 1985. Hepatopathology in experimental aflatoxicosis in chickens. Indian J. Anim. Sci. **55** (8) : 629-632.

Muller, R.D. C.W. Carlson. G. Scnenimick and G.S. Marchfield, 1970. The response of chicks, ducklings, gooslings, pheasants and poults to graded levels of aflatoxicosis. Poult. Sci. **49** (4) : 1346-1350.

Peckham, J. C., B. Doupnik and O. H. Jones. 1971. Acute toxicity of ochratoxins A and B in chicks. Appl. Microbiol. 21 : 492-494.

Peckham, M.C. 1975. Poisons and toxins. Disease of poultry. Ed. Hofstad, M.S., B.W. Calnek, C.F. Helmoldt. W.W. Reid and H.W. Yadev, Jr. (1975). 6th edn. 1977. Oxford and IBH Publishing Co., India, pp. 1134-1140.

Pohjanvirta, R., L. Sihvonen, and E. Karpanen. 1984. suspected sterigmatocystin toxicosis in poultry. Vet. Bull. 54 (7) : 4241 (Abstr.)

Thaxton , P., H.T. Tung and P.B. Hamilton. 1974. Immunisuppression in chicken by aflatoxin. Poultry Sci. 53 : 721.

Tung. H.T., J.W. Smith and P.B. Hamilton. 1971. Aflatoxicosis and bruising in the chicken. Poult Sci. 50 (3) : 795.

Threon, J.J., K.J., Vandermerwl, N. Liebenberg, H.J. B. Joubert and W. Nel. 1965. Acute liver injury in ducklings and rats as a result of ochratoxin poisoning. J. Pathol. Bacteriol. 91 (2) : 521 - 529.

Tuckler, T.L. and P.B. Hamilton. 1971. The effect of ochratoxin in broilers, Poultry. Sci. 50 (5) : 1637 (Abstr.)

Tapia, M.O., J.A. Lopez and A.P. Casaro, 1980. Aflatoxicosis in broiler fowl. Poult Abst. 7 (7) : A. No. 1903.

Venzytveld. W.A., D. C. Kelley and Dennis, 1970. Aflatoxicosis. The presence of aflatoxins ir their metabolites in livers and skeleton muscles of chickens. Poult Sci. 49 (4) : 1350-1356.

Wong, Z.A. and D.P.H. Hsieh. 1980. Comparative metabolism and toxicokinetics of aflatoxin B_1 in the monkey, rat and mouse. Toxical, Appl. Pharmacol. 55 : 115.

Yadgiri, B. 1970. Aflatoxins toxicity in different sps of animals (cited from A.R. Reddy, M.V Sc. thesis submitted to APAU, 1980).

Yoon, H.T. 1983. Studies on the toxicity of sterigmatocystin. Korean J. Vet. Pub. Health. 7 (2) : 85-91.

Vender Merwe, K.J., P.S. Steyn and L. Fourie. 1965a. Mycotoxins Part II. The constitution of ochratoxin, B and c metabolites of Aspergillus ochraceus. Cited by H. Chowdhury, C.W. Carlson and G. Semeniuk (1971). A study of ochratoxin toxicity in hens. Poultry Sci. **6** : 1855-1859.

CHAPTER

8

POSSIBILITIES AND LIMITATIONS OF DIAGNOSIS OF MYCOTOXICOSIS

A. Rajan
Director, Centre of Excellence in Pathology, College of Veterinary & Animal Sciences, Mannuthy, Trichur.

Mycotoxicosis has emerged as an important problem of economic importance as far as livestock industry is concerned. Different types of mycotoxins have been incriminated with livestock and poultry diseases. Among the toxins so far recognized aflatoxin continues to be the most common single mycotoxin which is ubiquitous in feed commodities. Aflatoxin contamintion is widely prevalent and there is need to monitor its presence and evaluate its economic importance in livestock health. A systematic approach identifying and quantifying common mycotoxins must be launched as a package of practices for animal health.

Mycotoxicosis can be diagnosed by various approaches. Examination of the feed commodity is resorted to as an indirect method of diagnosis. Various methods have been developed for this during the last two decades. The feed analysis has got its own limitations.

1. The feed samples taken may not be representative. Certain areas may have higher concentration (hot spots) than others. Toxin distribution may not be uniform.
2. When TLC is used and fluorescence is screened and analysed for mycotoxins, other fluorescent substances may interfere.
3. The incriminated feed might have been changed by the time the symptoms are manifested.
4. Contamination may occur at different stages. During growth, storage at factories, in retail shops and at farmers place of storage. At every stage, the feed has to be analysed. A factory cleared feed may still be positive at the feeding time.
5. Different mycotoxins may be present in the same feed and if only looked in for others will be missed.

Thin layer chromatography (TLC) is the most commonly

employed method. An efficient extraction and clean up are critical for successful TLC analysis. Several basic problems have contributed to variability and lack of precision in this method. Unawareness of sources of error, variability in extract clean-up techniques, sample extract application, differences in performance of the different instruments etc. are some of them.

The techniques employed in TLC have been changing rapidly and the preferred method now employed is high performance liquid chromatography. This system has all the techniques to improve performance like multidimensional approach and totally instrumentalised TLC. With new instrumentation, better precision and accuracy low determination limits are becoming possible. Of late GLC and Mass spectroscopy have been advocated.

The above, although, exhibits high sensitivity, requires sophisticated instrumentation. Therefore, the tests can be performed only in few well-established laboratories. But the need now is to have simple techniques, which could be used, at the field level. It is gratifying to note that diagnostic kits are being developed to meet this demand.

Diagnosis based on serology

The immunological analysis has better precision and specificity. Antibodies have been developed against AFBI, AFMI and DA. This has been exploited for diagnostic purposes. Aflatoxin has been detected in blood, cord blood, milk, meat and other tissues. It was shown by aflatoxin got excreted in milk and urine within first 48 h after consumption of cured aflatoxin. Maximum faecal excretion was noted from 1.5 to 3.5 days/post oral dosing. oral administration of mixed aflatoxin in lactating cows resulted in maximum excretion through mil (AFMI), faeces (AFBI) and urine by 24 h. Therefore, these material are good biosamples for aflatoxin analysis.

Aflatoxin in low levels in pig urine was detected by HPC and reflectance fluorodensitometry. The pigs were fed B_1, 1.7 ug and G_1, 2 ug/kg body weight for 16 weeks and B_1 and G_1 were detected at 0.05-0.39 ug and 0.14-15.8 uml respectively. A definite diagnosis of aflatoxicosis in animals, should therefore, rely entirely on the demonstration of the causative toxins in the excreta and tissues of the effected animals. Ho (1986) with the TLC clean-up and RF denstometry was able to detect aflatoxin at the lowest level (0.33 ug/ml).

It has been reported that animals as well as man excrete aflatoxin and their metabolites in urine following dietary exposure to such toxins. Sensitive methods like fluorodensitometry was able to detect B1 and M1 at concentrations as low as 0.14 ug and 0.34 ug respectively per ml of urine of the growing pigs.

Biological assay systems which are time consuming and not very preise, were in vogue for assay of aflatoxins. But these have been given up and chemical methods with precision have replaced these tests.

The presence of various types toxins in the same feed and their sinergistic effects have to be taken note of. The particular toxin when present in small quantities may not have any adverse effect but its effect will be amplified. Therefore effort should be to detect all common toxins.

Although many methods are available, limitations are many. Still an ideal method of diagnosis of mycotoxicosis remains to be identified and prescribed.

Summary

Detection and quantification of mycotoxins as aids in the diagnosis of mycotoxicosis have to be done in a systematic manner. Various diagnostic techniques have been described and immunologically based diagnostic tests have given promising results. HPLC gives satisfactory results in the laboratories. There are many limitations in employing these tests for diagnosis, these have been pointed out.

Suggestions for further reading

Ho *et al.* (1985). Determination of low levels of aflatoxin in the pig urine. J. Chi. Soc, Vet Sci., 11 : 9-16.

Jatlinek *et al.* 1989 Worldwide occurrence of mycotoxins in foods and feed. JAOC, 72 : 223-230.

Morgan, M.R.A. 1989. Mycotoxin immunoassays. Tetrahedron. 45 (8).

Proc, Int, Nat. Smyp. on Agricultural and Biological Aspects of Aflatoxin Related Health Hazards, Delhi. 1989. Delhi University.

Rodricks, J. 1977. Mycotoxins in human and animals health. Pathotox Publishers Inc., Illinois.

Shank, R.G. 1978. Mycotoxins and N-nitrosocompounds. CRC Reviews, Vol. II.

CHAPTER

9

THE INFLUENCE OF DIETARY PROTEIN, FAT, VITAMINS, MINERALS AND ANTIBIOTICS ON AFLATOXICOSIS IN POULTRY

V.R. Reddy,
Department of Poultry Science, College of Veterinary Science,
APAU, Hyderabad - 500 030

SYNOPSIS

The influence of dietary protein, fat, vitamins, minerals and antibiotics on aflatoxicosis. Higher protein in diet had a protective effect on aflatoxicosis and also increased the minimum effective dose. Lysine exacerbated the effects weight gain in aflatoxin-supplemented diets. Higher levels of fat in diet independent of degree of unsaturation reduced mortality during aflatoxicosis. Improved growthrate, however, was related to degree of unsaturation. Vitamin A deficiency in some experiments and thiamine deficiency had a protective effect against aflatoxicosis. Riboflavin or Vitamin D_3 deficiency made chickens sensitive to levels of aflatoxin too small to influence their growth rate. Vitamin mixtures failed to show beneficial effects in fatty live syndrome by aflatoxicosis Selenium and aureomycin did have a protective effect against aflatoxin toxicity.

Aflatoxins in diet of poultry cause depression in production, reduced feed intake, increased susceptibility to infectious diseases and mortality and the severity of aflatoxicosis in related to dose and duration of intake of aflatoxins within a flock. Alterations in the content of certain nutrient i.e., proteins, amino acids, fat, minerals, vitamins and antibiotics, in the diet of poultry are having an effect on aflatoxicosis in poultry.

Protein

It is reported that diets low in protein increases the severity of aflatoxicosis in rats (Modhavan and Gopalan, 1965 : McLean and Mclean, 1967), pigs (Sisk and Carlton, 1972), monkeys (Madhavan *et al.*, 1965) and chickens (Marcos and Lebshtein, 1963). That the higher dietary protein is having a protective effect on aflatoxicosis in chicken was shown (Table 1) by Smith *et al.* (1971). Increasing the dietary protein to a high level of 30% alleviated the effects of aflatoxicosis. Smith *et al.* (1971) opined that the protective effect of high protein in associated with overcoming the hypoproteinemia which develops in chicken during aflatoxicosis (Brown and Abrams, 1965).

Table 1. Influence of dietary protein level on the body weights of broilers at 28 d age in aflatoxicosis

	Body weight (g)		
Protein %	**Control**	**Aflatoxin ppm)**	**(5 % of Control**
10	180	137	76.1
20	318	254	79.9
30	389	368	94.6

Richardson *et al.* (1987a) observed that the minimum effective dose (MED) for inhibiting growth of chicken at 10, 12.75 and 15% protein was between 2 and 4 ug/g. The MED was increased to between 4 and 8 ug/g with increase in dietary protein to 20 and 25%. Liver weight and liver lipids had the same MED as that for body weight at protein levels from 10 to 25% except for the liver lipds at 10% protein. In further studies. Richardson *et al.* (1978a) observed that the enhanced effect of aflatoxin at low protein in diet is associated with a lower apparent MED and increased slope of response curves. The apparent MED (ug/g) at 10 and 12.75% protein diets respectively was 1.21 and 2.00 for body weight. 1.08 and 1.65 for liver lipids and 1.45 and 2.34 for liver relative weight.

Amino acids

Aflatoxin did not alter the digestibility of protein or absorption of amino acids. Lysine exacerbated the effect of aflatoxin, although it increased N retention to a level still below that with the basal diet. Methionine addition in the form of meat and feather meal improved appetite and increased weight gain in aflatoxin supplemented diets (Kryukov *et al.*, 1984).

Fat

The quantity as well as quality of dietary fat is having an effect on aflatoxicosis. The results obtained with turkey poults (Hamilton *et al.*, 1972) on inclusion of dietary fat in diets having aflatoxins are reproduced in Table 2.

Table 2. Effect of dietary fat on body weight, mortality, organ weights and lipids in liver and serum during aflatoxicosis in turkey poults.

Aflatoxin ppm	Dietary Fat%		
	2	6	18
	Body weight		
0	425	458	416
1	315	351	301
	Mortality		
0	4/40	3/40	4/40
1	10/40	11/40	2/40
	Liver weight, g/100 g body wt		
0	3.4	3.3	3.2
1	2.5	2.6	2.7
	Bursa weight, g/100 g body wt.		
0	0.14	0.14	0.14
1	0.11	0.11	0.13
	Liver Lipid, mg/100 mg dry liver		
0	14.8	12.8	14.6
1	17.0	16.7	19.1
	Serum lipids, mg/100 ml serum		
0	836	822	919
1	592	595	747
	Phospholipids, mg/100 ml serum		
0	226	271	222
1	59	71	148

Hamilton *et al.* (1972)

The dietary fat has an unusual effect on manifestation of aflatoxicosis in poults. The body weight during aflatoxicosis is not affected by fat from 2 to 18% but the high fat diet had an ameliorating effect against the mortality of aflatoxicosis. Liver weight and liver lipid were not influenced by dietary fat. Bursa weight regressed with aflatoxin indiet and high fat diet almost restored it to normal value. High liver of dietary fat (18%) restored serum lipid values to almost normal level and improved serum phospho lipids in aflatoxic poults.

Smith *et al.* (1971) tested the effect of 2, 6 and 16% dietary fat added in the form of cottonseed oil. Fat level did not influence growth rate (Fig. 1). The relative weight of liver and spleen were higher and that of bursa was lower with aflatoxin in diet. Supplemental fat increased the relative weight of liver but not of spleen and the effect on bursa was variable (Fig. 2). A striking effect was observed on mortality. Higher level of fat reduced mortality to a level that observed on aflatoxin free diet (Fig. 3).

The effect of quality of fat aflatoxicosis is shown in Table 3. Lipids appear to have a mortality sparing effect which does not depend on the degree of unsaturation and which does not appear to be the result of decreased absorption of aflatoxin from the intestinal tract. The other is a promotion of growth rate which is correlated with the degree of unsaturation of the dietary lipid since a high level of coconut oil or animal fat which are the low in unsaturated fatty acids did not promote growth while a high liver olive oil or safflower oil which are high in unsaturates promoted growth (Smith *et al.*, 1971).

Table 3. Effects of different dietary lipids on aflatoxicosis broilers.

Fat		Body weight at 3 wks (g)	Mortality
Olive oil	2%	211	24/50
	16%	263	10/50
Safflower oil	2%	325	16/50
	16%	422	0/50
Coconut oil	2%	212	27/50
	16%	237	3/50
Animal fat	2%	347	22/50
	16%	347	0/50

(Smith *et al.*, 1971)

Vitamins

Aflatoxicosis in chicken lowered Vitamin A but additional vitamin A did not result in decreased mortality (Kriz, 1970). Bryden *et al.* (1979) observed that the aflotoxin at 0.5 and 2.0 mg/kg diet failed to depress the growth in avitaminotic chicken. But aflotoxin at levels above 1 mg/kg diet efficiency when these birds received '8 mg retional/kg diet. Yen and Hamilton (1979) also reported that in chicken fed with aflatoxin contaminated diet, vitamin A deficiency improved growth, reduced mortality and prevented any effect on spleen, pancreas, gizzard, heart and liver size, serum protein serum cholesterol and serum uric acid but enhanced hypertrophy of preventriculous. They also reported severe decrease in Vitamin A content of serum and liver during aflatoxicosis in birds fed either sufficient or deficient in Vitamin A.

Vidwan Reddy *et al.*(1989) found no interaction in broiler chicks between dietary vitamin A (0,2000, 10,000 and 1,00,000 IU/kg) and aflatoxin (0,0.5, 2 ppm) in serum cholesterol. Liver Vitamin A decreased with increasing levels of aflotoxin. Serum cholesterol was, however, reduced in diet with 2 ppm aflatoxin and 0.1 million IU vitamin A per kg diet.

Todd *et al.* (1968) found that the addition of vitamin A, E and E to a commercial diet increased body weight gains of rats but did not influence the clinical signs, mortality and histopathological changes of aflatoxicosis in rats. Hamilton *et al.* (1974) reported that supplementing a diet adequate in vitamins with a four-fold excess of the NRC recommendations for vitamins afforded no protection against the growth inhibitory effect of aflatoxin in chicken (Table 4).

Diets deficient in riboflavin or vitamin D_3 made chicken sensitive to levels of aflatoxin too small to influence their growth rate (Table 4). In diets adequate in Vitamin D_3, aflatoxin reduced serum calcium levels by 20%. Vitamin K3 and vitamin E status had no influence on aflatoxicosis, as measured by growth rate (Table 4). A thiamine deficiency had a protective effect against the growth inhibitory effect of dietary aflatoxin. This unexpected protective effect can be rationalised on the basis that aflatoxin inhibits transport of fat from the liver while a thiamine deficiency stimulates fatty acid oxidation (Table 4) (Hamilton *et al.*, 1974).

Hamilton and Garlich (1971) observed that provision of 2.2 g choline chloride, 2.0 g inositol, 11 IU vitamin E and 13.2 ug vitamin

B_{12} per kg diet was without effect on aflatoxicosis in layers (aflatoxin 10 ug/g).

Table 4. Effect on body weight during aflatoxicosis of vitamins in chicks

Added vitamins	Aflatoxin, ug/g		
	0	0.625	5
All vitamins			
0	429[a]		252[b]
4 x NRC requirement	407[a]		252[b]
Control diet (7.9 ug riboflaving/g : 0.881 ICU vitamin D3/g)	397[c]	395[c]	
Riboflavin deficient (1.1 ug/g	138[a]	113[b]	
Vitamin D_3 deficient	174[d]	149[c]	
Vitamin E			
Control	399[a]		330[c]
Added Vitamin E (18 IU/kg)	467[b]		316[c]
Vitamin K_3			
Control	409[a]		307[c]
Normal (NRC requirement)	469[b]		306[c]
4 x Normal	456[b]		311[c]
Thiamine			
0.7 mg/kg	547[a]		634[b]
5.1 mg/kg	455[c]		415[d]

(Hamilton *et al.* 1974)

Minerals

Turkey poults were fed from 1 day to 5 weeks age, aflatoxin B_1 at 0.25 ug/g and selenium at 0.1, 5 or 10ug/g. Higher values in serum total protein, albumin, & globulin, B globulin and liver weights in poults fed aflatoxin B_1 and selenium indicated that selenium had a protective effect against aflatoxin toxicity (Table)(Burguera and Edds, 1983).

Table 5. Influence of selenium on body weight, liver weight and serum proteins during aflatoxicosis

	Selenium, ug/g			Aflatoxin, 0.25 ug/g selenium at ug/g		
	0.1	5	10	0.1	5	10
Body weight (g)	1408ab	1552a	1290ab	1417ab	1263ab	1360ab
Liver weight (g)	24.4b	270.0a	24.4b	24.1bc	16.0a	26.6a
In Serum						
Total protein (g/dI)	5.0a	5.3a	5.1a	4.8ab	5.2a	5.3a
Albumin, g/dI	2.82abc	3.45a	3.19a	3.22a	3.43a	3.53a
Globulin, g/dI	0.82a	0.88a	0.60a	0.48a	0.67a	0.66a
Globulin, g/dI	0.93ab	0.74abc	0.96a	0.78abc	0.71abc	0.83abc

(Burguera and Edss, 1983)

Antibiotics

In the experiments of Smith *et al.*(1971) aureomycin added to the aflatoxin diet improved body weight, feed conversion and reduced mortality (Table 6). The cause of these desirable effects in probably the inhibition of bacteria which are opportunistic invaders secondary to the debilitating effect of aflatoxin. Brown and Abrams (1965) were able to isolate Salmonella with increased frequency from birds with aflatoxicosis.

Table 6. Effect of aureomycin on aflatoxicosis is male broiler chicks (1 d to 21 d age)

	Body weight (g)	Feed conversion	Mortality
Control	363	1.73	0/50
Aureomycin (0.0055%)	360	1.75	0/50
Aflatoxin (10 ppm)	195	2.23	12/50
Aflatoxin (10 ppm) and Aureomycin (0.0055%)	211	1.98	6/50

(Smith *et al.*, 1971)

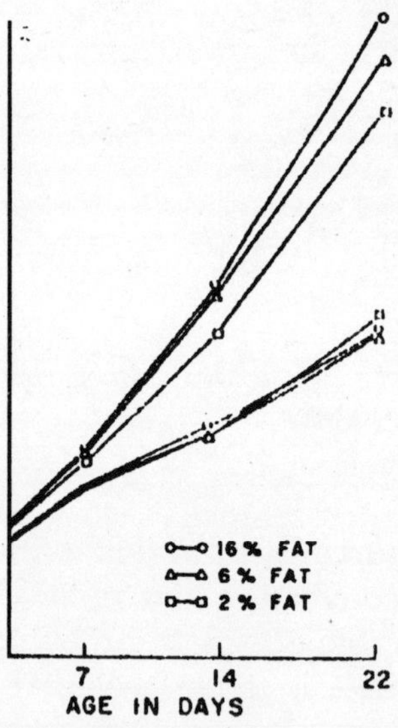

Fig. 1. Effect of dietry fat on body weight to afflatoxicosis. The diets contained to aflatoxin

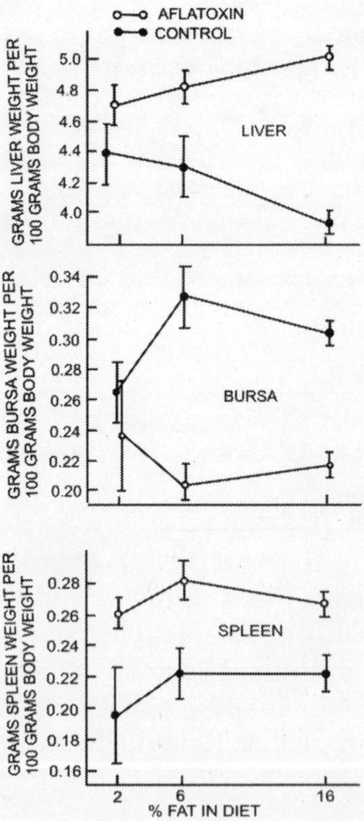

Fig. 2. Effect of dietary fat on liver, bursa and spleen response to aflatoxicosis. The diets contained 10 ppm aflatoxin vertical bars on the data points error of measns.

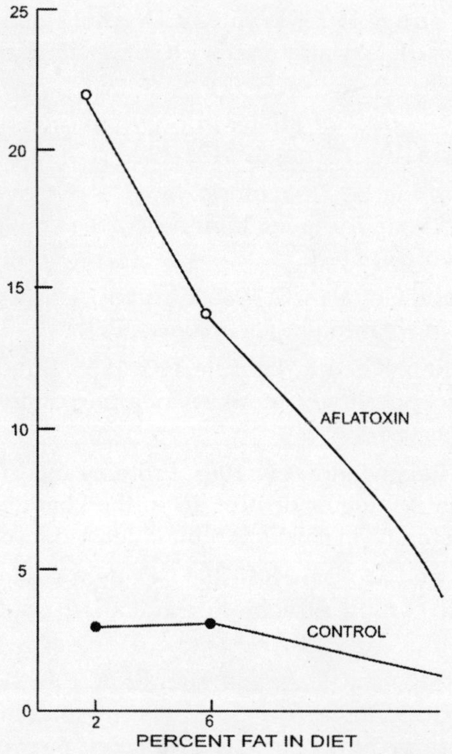

Fig. 3. Effct of dietary fat on mortality of aflatoxicosis. The diets contained 10 ppm aflatoxim

REFERENCES

Brown, J.M.M. and Abrams, L.1965. Biochemical studies on aflatoxicosis. Onderstepoort J. Vet. Res. 32 : 119-146.

Bryden, W.C., Cumming, R.B. and Balnave, D. 1979. the influence of vitamin A status on the response of chicken to aflatoxin B and changes in liver lipid metabolism associated with aflatoxicosis. British J. Nut, 41 : 529-540.

Burguera, J.A. and Edds, G.T. 1983. Influence on selenium on aflatoxin B or crotalaria toxicity in turkey poults. Am. J. Vet. Res. 44 : 1714-1717.

Hamilton, P.B., Garlick, J.D. 1972. Failure of vitamin supplementation to alter the fatty liver syndrome caused by aflatoxin. Poult Sci., 51 : 688-692.

Hamilton, P.B., Tung, H.T., Harris, J.R., Gainer, J.H. and Donaldson, W.E. 1972. The effect of dietary fat on aflatoxicosis in turkeys. Poults. Sci., 51 : 165-170.

Hamilton, P.B., Tung, H.T., Wyatt, R.D. and Donaldson, W.E. 1974. Interaction of dietary aflatoxin with some vitamin deficiencies. Poult Sci., 53 : 871-877.

Kriz. H. 1970. The effect of aflatoxin on vitamin A storage in livers of chickens. Acta. Vet. (Brno) 39 : 131-134.

Kryukov, V., Polunina, S., Zmachinskaya, G., Krivtsov, V. and Kalyagina, G. 1984. Effect of adding methionine to a feed mixture with aflatoxin. Ptitsevodstvo, 81 : 21-22.

Madhavan, T.V. and Gopalan, C. 1965. Effect of dietary protein on aflatoxin liver injury in weaning rats. Archieves Path. 80 : 123-126.

Madhavan, T.V. Rao, K.S. and Tulpule, P.G. 1965. Effect of dietary protein level on susceptibility of monkeys of aflatoxin liver injury. Indian J. Med. Res. 53 : 984-990.

Macroc, S.R. and Lebshetein, A.K. 1963. Proteins and toxicity : The effect of different dietary levels of protein in the changes produced by the "groundnut toxin" in chicks. Arabian Vet. Med. Assoc. J., 23 : 375-380.

McLean , A.E.M. and McLean, E.K. 1967. Protein depletion and toxic liver injury due to carbon tetrachloride and aflatoxin. Proc. Nut. Soc., 26 : 13.

Richardson, K.E., Nelson, L.A. and Hamilton, P.B. 1987a. Interaction of dietary protein level on dose response relationships during aflatoxicosis in young chickens. Poult. Sci., 66 : 969-976.

Richardson, K.E, Nelson, L.A. and Hamilton, P.B. 1987b. Effect of dietary fat level on dose response relationships during aflatoxicosis in young chickens. poult. Sci. 66 : 1470-1478.

Smith, J.W., Hill, C.H. and Hamilton, P.B. 1971. The effect of dietary modifications on aflatoxicosis in the broiler chicken. Poult. Sci., 50 : 768-774.

Sisk, D.B., and Carlton, W.W. 1972. Effect of dietary protein concentration on response of miniature swince to aflatoxins.

Todd, G.C., Shalkop, W.T. Dooley, K.L. and Wiseman, H.G., 1968. Effects of ration modification on aflatoxicosis in the rat. American J. Vet. Res., 29: 1855-1861.

Vidwan Reddy, K., Rao, P.V. and Ramasubba Reddy, V., 1989. Effect of aflatoxin on the performance of broiler chicks-fed diets supplemented with vitamin A. Indian J. Anim, Sci., 59 : 140-144.

Yen. C.C. and Hamilton, P.B. 1979. Interaction of vitamin A deficiency of aflatoxicosis. Poult. Sci. 58 : 1124.

CHAPTER

10 AFLATOXIN IN FEED STUFFS AND ITS EFFECT ON THE PERFORMANCE OF CHICKEN, QUAIL AND GUINEA FOWL

V.R. Sadagopan
Principal Scientist Project Directorate on Poultry Rajendranagar, Hyderabad - 500 030

Mycotoxicosis in the generic name given to the toxic syndrome, resulting from intake of feed stuffs infested with moulds and their metabolic products by animals and man. Mycotoxicosis have been known for a very long time, but only recently they have aroused much scientific interest particularly in poultry. During 1940s and 1950s, outbreak of mycotoxicosis occurred in the USA causing mortality in swine due to feeding of mouldy maize. But little efforts were made to elucidate the root cause of such disease until the outbreak of Turkey 'X' disease in England during 1960. The causative agent responsible for Turkey 'X' disease was later identified to be a mixture of toxins produced by some strains of *Aspergillus flavus* growing in groundnut meal fed to the affected birds. The heavy mortalities on poultry farms drastically changed the once-neglected disease into a practical problem. It is now considered that more than 200 toxic metabolites produced by moulds can cause mycotoxicosis in farm animals. Aflatoxin group of toxins may be one of the most significant pollutant, produced by *Aspergilus flavus* or *A. parasiticus.* During the last two decades or so scientific discoveries have emphasized the hazards of mycotoxins in animal and poultry production.

Aspergillus flavus is of worldwide distribution with wide range of substrate, temperature humidity, moisture and other condition for growth and production of aflatoxins. Aflatoxin consists of closely related chemical structured namely B_1, B_2, G_1, G_2, B_1 is the most toxic and carcinogenic and occur most commonly in the contaminated feed stuffs. Groundnuts, cotton, seeds, certain oilseeds and their products. Maize and a few other cereal grains and more susceptible to aflatoxin contamination. This is due to largely poor drying and storage practices during post-harvest periods. Preharvesting contamination also cannot be ruled out. Aflatoxicosis in poultry has been characterized by haemorrhage in many tissues, reduced growth rate, hepatotoxicosis anorexia, and decreased egg products in laying flock.

In our country systematic reporting of mycotoxicosis have not been attempted resulting in most of the case having gone undetected or unnoticed. It has been reported that all important Khaki Campbell ducks in India, which were distributed in various States have all diet mainly due to aflatoxicosis (Rao, 1968). Gopala and his associated (1968) reported incidence of aflatoxicosis in chicks in Mysore State wherein 2.210 chicks died within a period of one week. Aflatoxicosis outbreaks in commercially poultry farms around Chittor town of Andhra Pradesh were reported by Choudhry and Rao (1982) and Lakshmanachar (1982). During the early eighties a number of outbreaks occurred in Ranikhet in northern India despite proper vaccination with potent F_1 and R_SB vaccines and caused heavy loss to poultry farmers. The presence of higher levels of aflatoxin in poultry feeds has adversely affected the immunity of the flock. However, no analytical data has been given in support of the above trouble.

Indian work of the effects of aflatoxocosis in poultry

Brief Review

Earlier to the 1980s no evidence of systematic work on this area is available. Perhaps APAU was the first in the country to initiate research on various aspects of aflatoxicosis in 1979 and continued. In view of the severity of the outbreaks, a National Seminar on Aflatoxins was organized during October 1982 at Central Avian Research Institute, Izatnagar (UP). Subsequently intensive research on this area was started by CARI, INKV and by other research institutions and contributed significantly. The following is a brief account of the work conducted by different workers.

Subba Rao *et al.* (1977) showed that dietary level of 2000 PPB of aflatoxin is innocuous for growth in broilers. A series of investigations aflatoxicosis were initiated by APAU workers. Rajesekhar Reddy *et al.* (1982) tested graded doses of aflatoxin of 0.25, 0.50.0.75, 1.00 1.25 and 1.50 ppm on broilers (0-6 weeks age) and reported a decreased growth and feed consumption with 0.5 ppm onwards compared to control 0.25 ppm aflatoxin diet.

Significant increase in liver weight from 0.50 ppm. Kidney from 5 ppm, spleen from 1.50 ppm, and regression of bursa of fabricius from .25 ppm was reported. In another study significant dose-related reduction in performance of broilers (0-4 weeks) from 0.75 ppm aflatoxin level as noticed (Nandakumar Reddy *et al.*, 1984). In layers a significant education in hen-day egg production was noticed with 1.00 ppm although feed consumption was unaffected at 200 ppb level. In egg quality no difference was observed (Iqbal *et al.* 1983). In interaction of increased severity of vitamin A deficiency was noticed with 2 ppm dietary aflatoxin Vidwan Reddy *et al.* 1989).

In view of the need for more experimental evidences and conflicting exports available in literature, a series of investigations were carried out at CARI, Izatnagar. Studies were undertaken to find out the effect of commonly-occurring dietary aflatoxin levels on the performance of RIF x WL cross, White, Leghorn, Quail and Guinea Fowls to determine dietary aflatoxin levels which can be tolerated by these birds.

MATERIALS AND METHODS

In the laboratory, aflatoxin was produced by infesting rice with *Aspergillus parasiticus* (Shotwell *et al.*, 1966). The autoclaved, dried and powdered infested rice, which was estimated for aflatoxin content (Pons *et al.*, 1966) was used in place of maize to contain various levels of aflatoxin in the test diets of all the experiments.

In experiment 1. RIR x WL cross chicks: in experiment 2. WL chicks and in experiment 3. quail chicks were employed. Basal diet containing 23% crude protein and 2900 kcal. ME/kg for chicken and 27% protein with 2800 kcal. ME/kg for quails were formulated. In each experiment, five test diets were prepared by replacing yellow maize of basal diets with dried infested rice power as to obtain 0, 0.2, 0.3, 0.5 and 0.75 ppm level of aflatoxin. The basis for selecting the above toxin levels was the practical occurrence of aflatoxin in poultry feed stuffs normally. Trials with WL and WL X RIR cross chicks were conducted from 9 to 58 days of age. In both the trials day-old chicks were obtained, vaccinated, wing banded and maintained under standard conditions of brooding, feeding and watering for the first 8 days. At the start of the experiment on 8th day, the chicks were weighed individually, distributed randomly on uniform body weight basis into 15 groups of seven chicks each group. Three such groups wee offered the same test diet *ad. lib.*

In the third experiment day-old quail chicks were taken and maintained in battery brooder under standard feeding regime for 4 days. On 5th day the chicks were distributed into 15 groups of 24 chicks in each on equal body weight basis. Each test diet was offered to triplicate groups of chicks from 5th to 35th day. Feed and water were provided *ad. lib.* Nutritional balance studies were carried out from 44th to 46th days of age for quail. Diets and excreta from different balance trials were analyzed for chemical composition (AOAC, 1970) and aflatoxin content (Pons *et al.*, 1966). In the three trials, individual weekly body weight group feed consumption; feed efficiency and mortality were recorded. At the end of each trial, 2 chicks from each dietary treatment were taken randomly, scarified for gross pathological lesions in the organs. Hematological studies (Coles, 1974), serum protein content (Benjamin, 1961) and blood uric acid content (Oser, 1965) were carried out at the end of each trial using 6 chicks from each treatment.

In the fourth trial Guinea fowl keets were sued. A reference diet containing 275 crude protein and 2854 kcal ME/kg was formulated. Six test diets were prepared by including the infested rice in place of maize so as to get 0.0, 0.2, 0.3, 0.5, 0.75 and 1.00 ppm dietary aflatoxin level. One hundred and twenty day-old Guinea fowl keets from the same hatch were maintained in battery brooders on reference diet upto 24 days of age. On 25th day, they were weighted individually and distrubed into 12 groups on equal body weight basis so as to have six keets in each group. The groups were allotted randomly to one dietary treatment.

Experimental feeding was continued from 25 to 36 days of age. Feed and water were provided *ad lib.* Weekly individual body weight group feed consumption and were recorded. At the end of the experiment, 2 birds from each replicate of all the 6 treatments were sacrificed for gross pathological lesions if any. Data collected from all the experiments were analysed statistically (Snedecor and Cochran, 1967).

RESULTS AND DISCUSSION

Experiments 1, 2 and 3

Data on body weight, feed consumption feed gain ratio obtained in all the three experiments are shown in Table 1. It may be seen from the data that a significant depression both in body weight and feed consumption was noticed in White Leghorn and RIR x White Leghorn cross chicks at 58 days of age even at low level of 0.2 ppm aflatoxin content of the diet. The feed conversion remained unaffected from

0.2 to 0.5 ppm aflatoxin level respectively. The results obtained by other workers on the effect of dietary aflatoxin on the performance of chicks varied according to the dietary level of aflatoxin tested, duration of feeding, breed and strain used in the experiment supports the present observation (Smith and Hamilton, 1970; Tung *et al.*, 1971; Culvenor, 1974; Arafa *et al.*, 1981; Rajesekhar Reddy *et al.*, 1982; Ubosi *el al.*, 1985). However, in the present study a significant decrease in body weight was observed both in RIR x WL cross and White Leghorn chicks, even at 0.2 ppm level. On the other hand different dietary levels of aflatoxin on the performance of quail chicks indicated that growth of chicks fed on diets containing 0.2, 0.3 and 0.5 ppm were comparable with that of control diet. Dawron *et al.*(1977) and Wilson *et al.*(1987) reported that quails started showing signs of reduced body weight at 0.4 ppm level and above whereas Arafa *et al.* (1981) reported decrease in body weight only at 0.7 PPM. On the contrary. Sinha and Asrora (1987) reported a safe level of 1000 ppb in Hyline broilers. This needs further investigation.

Analysis of the data on body weight of cuinea fowls (Table 2) at 50 and 86 days of age indicated a non-significant difference between different dietary levels of aflatoxin and between the reference and aflatoxin diets. Dietary aflatoxin upto 1 ppm did not adversely influence the body weight, feed consumption and efficiency of feed utilization. Number of guinea fowls died during the experiments in different dietary treatments was within the normal limit and no mortality was attributable to the dietary aflatoxin content.

Feed consumption and feed efficiency

Data indicated (Table 1) a significant reduction in the feed consumption in RIR x WL cross chicks even at a low level of 0.2 ppm toxin. Efficiency of feed utilization in RIR x WL cross chicks was not influenced even upto 0.5 ppm level. Similar pattern was observed in White Leghorn chicks but at 0.5 ppm level the efficiency was reduced compared to other low level. However, in quail chicks the feed consumption remained unaffected upto 0.5 ppm level but feed efficiency of utilization was reduced at 0.5 and 0.75 ppm level. Reduced feed consumption due to toxin levels ranging from 0.4 to 0.7 ppm was also reported by other workers (Damron *et al.*, 1977 : Wilson *et al.*, 1978 and Alfafa *et al.*, 1981).

Nutrient retention

Results of balance studies on dry matter, protein, calcium and

Table 1. Mean body weight, feed consumption and feed/gain ratio of RIR x WL cross, WL and quail chicks given different dietary treatment

Attributes	Dietary aflatoxin levels (ppm)*				
	0.0	0.2	0.3	0.5	0.75
			RIR X WL cross chicks		
Body weight (g)	625.0[a]	546.0[b]	503.0[c]	454.0[d]	371.0[a]
(58th day)	±16.7	±16.0	±13.4	±13.8	±13.5
Feed consumption (g)	1576.0[a]	1353.0[b]	1266.0[b]	1235.0[b]	975.0[c]
(9-58 days)	±17.9	±38.9	±98.7	±13.8	±23.3
Feed/gain ratio	2.61[b]	2.63[b]	2.70[b]	2.99[ab]	3.55[a]
(9-58 days)	±0.00	±0.00	±0.00	±0.00	±0.00
			WL chicks		
Body weight (g)	612.0[a]	508.0[b]	507.0[b]	424.0[c]	339.0[d]
(58th day)	±13.3	±14.1	±12.0	±10.6	±17.0
Feed consumption (g)	1446.0[a]	1337.0[b]	1325.0[b]	1292.0[b]	1011.0[c]
(9-58 days)	±27.1	±16.5	±55.8	±27.3	±43.0
Feed/gain ratio	2.59[c]	2.86[bc]	2.91[b]	3.34[a]	3.55[a]
			Quail chicks		
(9-58 days)	±0.10	±0.10	±0.00	±0.10	±0.10
Body weight (g)	140.0[a]	136.0[a]	129.0[a]	123.0[ab]	113.0[b]
(35th day)	±2.5	±2.3	±2.4	±2.3	±2.5
Feed consumption (g)	401.0[a]	358.0[a]	371.0[a]	354.0[ab]	306.0[ab]
(5-35 days)	±1.5	±2.7	±4.2	±8.5	±15.1
Feed / gain ratio	3.08[b]	3.20[ab]	3.21[ab]	3.24[a]	3.26[a]
(5-35 days)	±0.00	±0.00	±0.10	±0.00	±0.10

*abc Values which do not share common letters in a row, are significantly different (P<0.5).

Table 2. Effect of different dietary level of aflatoxin on the performance of guinea fowls

Dietary treatment	Initial body weight at 25 days of age (g)	Body weight at 50 days of age (g)	Body weight at 86 days of age (g)	Feed consumption at 50 days of age (g)	Feed efficiency at 50 days at age (g)	Feed consumption at 86 days of age (g)	Feed efficiency at 86 days of age	Number of birds died
Reference	88.0±5.4	632.0±29.7	998.0±24.1	1,585±27.0	2.91±0.15	2,763±29.0	3.03±0.11	1 (12)
Aflatoxin B1								
0.2 ppm	89.0±5.7	653.0±33.0	1,025.0±15.4	1,531±14.0	2.71±0.24	2,621±27.0	2.80±0.29	2(12)
0.3 ppm	87.0±5.0	653.3±25.0	995.0±27.2	1,598±21.0	2.82±0.37	2,707±21.0	2.98±0.17	1(12)
0.5 ppm	86.0±5.4	639.0±23.0	1,004.0±20.3	1,565±26.0	2.83±0.16	2,850±31.0	3,10±0.18	1(12)
0.75 ppm	87.0±7.3	641.0±25.2	994.0±32.4	1,524±17.0	2.75±0.33	2,752±30.0	3.03±0.20	2(12)
1.00 ppm	87.0±6.6	631.0±21.6	993.0±27.0	1,519±31.0	2.79±0.22	2,650±35.0	2.92±0.09	1 (12)

1Number given in parentheses indicate the Number of guinea-fowls taken initially in the particular dietary treatment.

phosphorus retention obtained with RIR x WL cross, WL and quail chicks are given in Table 3. It is evident from the nutrient retention data that a progressive decrease in nutrient retention was recorded as the level of aflatoxin was raised. Even ppm dietary aflatoxin level significantly reduced the nutrient retention except calcium.

In WL chicks the trend was similar but noticed from 0.3 ppm level onwards. In quail also a similar trend was noticed. Reduced feed consumption and nutrient retention was attributable to the impairment of digestion and absorption due to the presence of aflatoxin in the diet. Similar findings were also reported by Osborne *et al.* (1976) was Huff *et al.* (1977).

Hematological studies

Dietary aflatoxin level on hematological values of RIR x WL, WL and quail are presented in Table 4. The PCV, hemoglobin content, RBC count and serum protein content were not influenced by tested levels of aflatoxin in RIR x WL, WL chicks except that a marked reduction in serum protein and an increase in blood urine acid at 0.75 level were noticed.

In quail chicks, the PCV and erythrocyte dietary aflatoxin levels did not affect counts. However, a decrease in hemoglobin and serum protein content was observed at 0.5 and 0.75 ppm levels.

Gross pathological lesions and mortality

Gross pathological lesions observed in sacrificed RIR x WL cross chicks were mild enlargement of liver with granularity on surface in 2 birds at 0.2 ppm level. At 0.3 ppm level the liver was enlarged. pale and had haemorrhagic streaks. The lesions in the liver at 0.5 level were similar to those observed at 0.3 ppm. haemorrhages and granularity of the surface of liver was more marked at 0.75 ppm level. Mild enlargement of kidney and haemorrhages on its surface was found in chicks above 0.3 ppm level. No change in the bursa fabricius was observed.

In WL chicks enlargement and pale discolouration of live was noticed at 0.2 and 0.3 ppm levels. Haemorrhages were more marked with granularity of liver surface at 0.5 ppm level. At 0.75 ppm level, liver, kidney were pale with hemorrhagic foci and marked streaks without any enlargement.

In quail chicks, pale liver at 0.2 ppm level, pale and slight enlarged liver at 0.3 ppm, pale discolouration of liver without appreciable

Table 3. Effect of different dietary levels of aflatoxin on dry matter, protein, calcium and phosphorus retention in RIR x WL cross, WL and quail chicks

Dietary aflatoxin	Dry-matter retention*	Protein retention*	Calcium retention*	Phosphorus retention*
		RIR x WL cross chicks		
0.00	70.43±0.8[a]	17.60±1.2[a]	0.68±0.0[a]	0.29±0.0[a]
0.2	63.22±1.2[b]	15.68±0.6[b]	0.66±0.1[a]	0.23±0.0[b]
0.3	56.67±2.3[b]	14.10±1.5[c]	0.56±0.1[b]	0.22±0.0[b]
0.5	57.50±0.6[b]	13.84±0.8[cd]	0.58±0.1[b]	0.22±0.0[b]
0.75	49.78±0.0[c]	12.33±1.3[d]	.49±0.0[c]	0.19±0.0[c]
		WL chicks		
0.0	68.50±2.5[a]	17.12±0.3[a]	0.66±0.0[a]	0.28±0.0[a]
0.2	62.50±0.5[a]	15.52±0.0[a]	0.65±0.0[a]	0.23±0.0[b]
0.3	49.50±1.3[b]	12.34±0.8[b]	0.49±0.1[b]	0.19±0.0[c]
0.5	46.80±0.0[b]	11.27±0.1[bc]	0.47±0.0[b]	0.17±0.1[c]
0.75	43.00±0.0[b]	10.67±0.0[c]	0.43±0.0[c]	0.17±0.1[c]
		Quail chicks		
0.0	30.32±1.3[a]	8.82±0.1[a]	0.34±0.0[a]	0.15±0.0[a]
0.2	27.91±0.2[a]	8.19±0.0[a]	0.32±0.0[a]	0.14±0.0[a]
0.3	21.85±0.7[b]	6.35±0.4[b]	0.25±0.0[b]	0.11±0.0[b]
0.5	21.28±0.0[b]	6.18±0.0[b]	0.24±0.0[b]	0.10±0.0[b]
0.75	21.57±0.0[b]	6.27±0.0[b]	0.24±0.0[b]	0.11±.0.0[b]

[a'b'c] Values which do not share common letters in a column are significantly different ($p<0.5$).

*, g/chick/3 days

Table 4. Effect of dietary aflatoxin on haematological values of RIR x WL cross, WL and quail chicks

Aflatoxin level in diet (ppm)	Packed-cell volume (%)	Haemoglobin (g/100 ml)	Erythrocyte count (x $10^6/mm^3$)	Serum protein (g/100 ml)	Blood* uric acid (mg/100 ml)
			RIR x WL cross chicks		
0.0	25.0	7.00	2.35	5.50[a]	8.4[b]
0.2	28.0	6.72	2.59	5.10[a]	8.0[b]
0.3	27.0	6.11	2.42	5.20[a]	7.8[b]
0.5	26.0	6.16	2.20	5.00[a]	6.9[b]
0.75	26.0	5.99	2.42	3.99[b]	11.0[a]
			WL chicks		
0.0	30.0	7.24	2.47	6.28[a]	6.7[b]
0.2	31.0	8.15	2.58	5.88[a]	7.0[b]
0.3	33.0	7.88	2.68	6.00[a]	7.5[b]
0.5	29.5	6.81	2.59	5.60[b]	6.2[b]
0.75	29.5	7.0	2.42	4.12[b]	9.0[a]
			Quail chicks		
0.0	44.5	8.24	2.94	3.38	-
0.2	45.0	7.06	2.86	4.50	-
0.3	47.5	7.06	2.87	4.00	-
0.5	45.0	6.74	2.91	4.00	-
0.75	44.5	6.83	2.97	3.25	-

*Blood uric acid in quails was not estimated.

[a'b'c'] Values which do not share common letters in a column, are significantly different (P<0.5).

enlargement at 0.5 ppm level were noticed. At 0.75 ppm level liver and kidney were pale and in few birds orange were enlarged.

Mortality attributable to dietary aflatoxin occurred in RIR x WL cross 9.0%; quail chicks 11.2 % at 0.75 ppm level. In WL chicks 9.52 per cent mortality was recorded at both 0.5 and 0.75 ppm levels. In these trails no traces of aflatoxin was detected in muscles of the birds received different levels of aflatoxin.

SUMMARY

Experiments were conducted to study the effect of graded levels of (induced) dietary aflatoxin on the performance of various categories of poultry and permissible dietary level of aflatoxin. White Leghorn chicks, RIR x WL cross, quail chicks and Guinea fowl keets were exmployed in the study. Dietary aflatoxin levels of , 0.2, 0.3, 0.5 and 0.75 ppm are tested in chicken and quail. In addition to the above levels, .00 ppm was also tested in guinea fowl. Details of the experiments with criteria considered for evaluation were described in the text. Significant reduction in the performance of White Leghorn and cross of RIS WL chicks, was noticed even at the lowest level of 0.2 ppm dietary aflatoxin level. On the other hand, the performance of quail chicks received diets containing 0.2 and 0.3 ppm toxic was comparable with control group. However, retention of nutrients was adversely affected at 0.3 ppm and above. Reduction in serum protein content was observed at 0.75 ppm level of White Leghorn and RIR x WL cross chicks. Guinea fowls were found to be the most resistant to the dietary aflatoxin upto 1 ppm level tested.

REFERENCES

AAOC. 1970. Official Methods of Analysis. XI Edition.. Association of Analytical Chemists, Washington DC.

Arafa, A.S., Bloomer, R.J., Wilson, H.R., Simpson, C.F. and Harmes. R.H. 1981. British Poultry Science, 22 : 431-36.

Benjamin, M.N. 1961. Outline of Veterinary Clinical Pathology. II Edu., Iowa State University Press, Ames, Iowa.

Coles, H.E. 1974. Veterinary Clinical Pathology. II Edn., W.B. Saunders Company, Philadelphia and London.

Culvenor, C.C.J. 1974. Australian Veterinary Journal, 50 : 69-78.

Choudhry, C.H. and Rao, M.R.K. 1982. Poultry Advisor, XIV : 75-76.

Damron, B.L., Manly, J.G., Wilson, H.R. and Harms, R.H. 1977. Poultry Science, 56 : 1708.

Gopal, T., Sayed Zaki, Narayanaswamy and Premlata, S. 1968. Indian Veterinary Journal , 46 : 348-49.

Huff, W.E., Chang, C.F., Garlich, J.D. and Hamilton, P.B. 1977. Poultry Science, 56 : 1724.

Iqbal, Q.K., Rao, P.V. and Reedy, S.J., 1983. Indian Journal of Animal Science, 53 : 1277.

Lakshmanachar, N., Parameshwar Rao, Inayatulla Khan, Ramalingeswar, D. 1982. Poultry Advisor, XVI, 57-58.

Laxmirajam, S. 1982. Indian Journal of Animal Sciences, 54: 348-52.

Nandakumar Reddy, D., Rao, P.V., Reddy, V.R. and Badgiri, B. 1984. Indian Journal of Animal Science, 54 : 68.

Osborne, D.J., Huff, W.E. and Hamilton, P.B. 1976. Poultry Science, 55 : 2075.

Oser, B.L. 1965. Hawk's Physiological Chemistry, 14th Edn., McGraw Hill Book Company, London.

Pons W.A., Cacullu, A.F., Lee, L.S., Robertson, J. A., Franz A. O. and Goldblatt, L. A., 1966. Journal of the Association of Official Analytical Chemistry, 49 : 405-10.

Rajesekhar Reddy, A., Reddy, V.R., Rao, P.V. and Yadagiri, B., 1982. Indian Journal of Animal Science, 52 : 405-410.

Rao, S.B.V. 1968. Indian Poultry Gazette. 52 : 1

Shotwell, O. L., Hesseltine, C.W., Stubbefield, R. D. and Sorenson, W. G. 1966. Appl. Microbiol. 14 : 425.

Sinha, R.B.P. and Aroro, S.P. 1987. Indian Journal of Animal Nutrition 4(1) : 12-19.

Smith, J.W. and Hamilton, P.B. 1970. Aflatoxicosis in the Broiler chicken. Poultry Science, 49 : 207-15.

Snedecor, G.W. and Cochran, W.G. 1967. Statistical methods, 6th Edn. Iowa State University Press, Ames, Iowa.

Subha Rao, I.V.R., Singh, K.S., Tripathi, R.K. and Rao, B.S. 1977. Indian Journal of Poultry Sciences, 12 : 42-48.

Tung, H.T., Smith, J.W. and Hamilton, P.B. 1971. Poultry Science 50 : 795-99.

Bosi, C.O., Hamilton, P.B., Dunnington, E.A. and Siegel, P.B. 1985. Poultry Science, 64 : 1065-70.

Idwan Reddy, K., Rao, P.V. and Reddy, V.R. 1989. Indian Journal of Animal Science, 59 : 140-144.

Ison, H.R., Manley, J.G., Harmes, R. H. and Damron, B. C. 1978. Poultry Science, 57 : 403-407.

CHAPTER

11

EFFECT OF DIETARY AFLATOXIN ON THE PERFORMANCE OF COMMERCIAL AND BROILER CHICKEN

Dr. A. Rajesekher Reddy
Assistant Professor AICRP on Poultry for Eggs, Rajendranagar, Hyderabad-30

ABSTRACT

Aflatoxins are fungal metabolites elaborated by *Aspergillus* sps. Aflatoxin depressed growth of broilers as low as 0.5 ppm. Mortality was observed at 1 ppm aflatoxin. The visceral organs like liver, kidney were target organs for aflatoxin. Fat metabolism was deranged at 0.75 ppm effecting fatty livers. Some of the biochemical parameters like serum proteins, serum chlolesterol, serum uric acid were decreased. The increased lysosomal enzyme activity was responsible for the bruise formation in muscles. Aflatoxinssuppressed the growth of immunologicalorgans like bursa of fabricius and thymus. Possibility of carryover of aflatoxin B1 metabolite like M_1 into muscles and livers was lives was evident. Lowered haeatological value such as PCV, Hb, RBC together with splenomegaly at about 1.5 ppm and above levels of aflatoxin suggest that aflatoxicosis induce haemolytic anemia. Pathological changes noted in the effected birds were enlarged and smooth livers with greyish discolouration, enlarged injected kidneys and atrophy of bursa of fabricius. Histopathology of birds revealed fatty changes in liver, tubular degeneration in kidney and lymphoid depletion with fibrosis in the bursa. Dietary aflatoxin in a range of 0.25 to 0.5 ppm could be safe level in diets for broilers.

Aflatoxins are fungal metabolites elaborated on various feed ingredients when contaminated with *Aspergillus* sps. These fungi are mainly *A. flavus* and *A. parasiticus* and produces aflatoxin B_1, B_2 and G_1 and G_2. *A. parasiticus* predominantly produce aflatoxin B_1, Aflatoxins contain lactone rings with coumarin nucleus. B_2 and G_2 are dihydro derivatives of B_1 and G_1. G_1 contains extra coumarin structure. These fractions can be classified as B_1 G_1 B_2 G_2 based on their decreased order of toxicity.

Aflatoxins are hepatotoxic and nephrotoxic agents. Besides this, they are carcinogenic. Mutagenic and teratogenic effects of aflatoxin have been studied (Chu, 1977)

The susceptibility of birds of aflatoxin B_1 is found to vary with species. The maximum safe levels of aflatoxin in the diets of ducklings/man, chicken, pigs, cattle and sheep were reported as 0.03, 0.20, 0.2 to 0.3, 0.3 to 0.6 and 1.75 ppm respectively (Kumar and Gowdaveeranarayana, 1977). Among various breeds, the Brahma was the most susceptible to aflatoxin while the Plymouth Rock was the most resistant to aflatoxin (Rivelli *et al.*, 1969).

Although India has a considerable poultry population, reported outbreaks of aflatoxicosis in poultry as a few (Gopal *et al.*, 1969 and Rao *et al.*, 1985). The incidence of sporadic cases of aflatoxicosis poisoning are very common. In many instances the outbreaks were not confirmed because of lack of aflatoxin analytical facilities in feed and also interaction with many more mycotoxins. During the last 10 years, considerable work on aflatoxin poultry has been carried on in India particularly in the Department of Poultry Science, A.P.Agricultural University. The primary objective of these studies have been to know the maximum safe levels of aflatoxins in diets for broilers.

Metabolism of aflatoxin

Aflatoxin molecule biodegrades into at least six ways (Fig. 1).

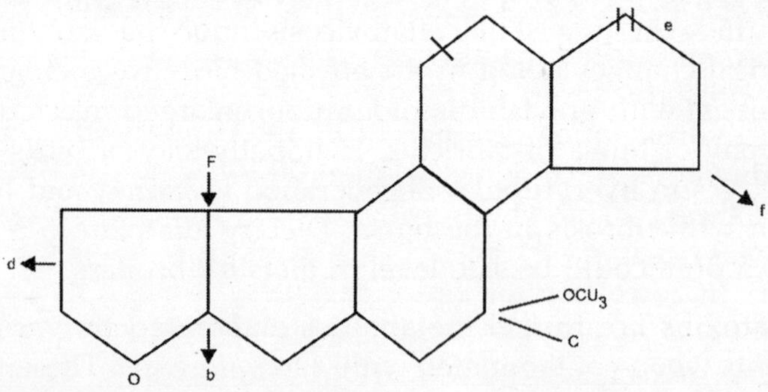

a) Reduction of venyl ether double bond
b) Opening of bisfuranoid structure
c) 0-demethylation
d) Hydrolytic fission of coumarin lactone
e) Cyclopentenone reduction
f) Hydroxylation

Fig. 1. Aflatoxin molecule

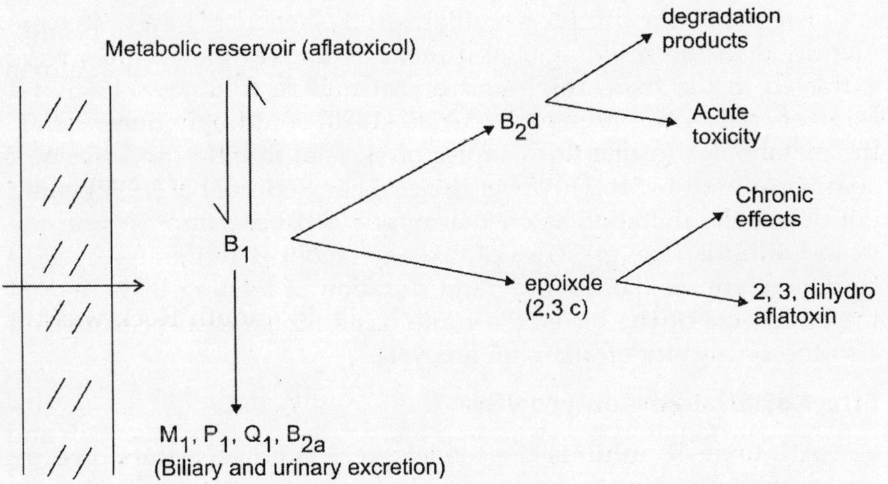

Fig.2 A diagramatic representation of the metabolism and mechanism of action of aflatoxin B_1 showing uptake by liver cell, its conversion to six metabolites and probable roles of B_{2a} and the epoxide as the acute and chronic toxins respectively.

These are (a) reduction of venyl ether double bond i.e. aflatoxin B_1 and G_1 are converted into aflatoxin B_2 and G_2. The double bond is important for the toxicity. (b) Cyclopentenone reduction i.e. aflatoxin B_1 and B_2 are converted into aflatoxicol and dihydro aflatoxicol respectively. This conversion takes places in cytosol. (c) Hydroxylation 2 hydroxlation compound i.e. aflatoxin B_{2a}. It is hemiacetal compound formed in the presence of microsomal enzymes and is responsible for the acute toxicity by means of non-specific inhibition of liver enzymes. (d) B_{2a} can also further metabolized into degradation products i.e. by opening of bisfuranoid structure of aflatoxin (at 20 c position). Theother hydroxylation products of B_1 are M_2 (4 hydroxylation), Q1 (22 hydroxylation). (e) 0-demethylation, (at 16th c position) of aflatoxin B_1 i.e. aflatoxin P_1. These hydroxylation productsof afla B_1 are present in biliary, or urinary excretion as it is or in conjugated form. (f) hydrolytic fission of coumarin structure i.e. aflatoxin B_1 coumaric acid. This product is achieved by boiling an aqueous solution of the toxin. The coumarin structure is essential for the induction of the acute liver.

The chronic effects of aflatoxin B_1 are manifested by the product of aflatoxin B_1, 2,3 epoxide which is metabolically active in the liver. This product is known as proximal carcinogen, and is responsible for the carcinogenicity in different species. It also reacts with cellular nucleophiles such as nucleic acid, protein and SH group compounds.

The metabolic products of aflatoxin B_1 such as M1 and M2 were identified in the milk, eggs and meat. Aflatoxin metabolites were extracted in the liver, thigh and breast muscle (Platnow, 1965 and Mratzer *et al.*, 1969). Venzytveld *et al.* (1970) could only demonstrate the metabolites in one third saples of skeletal muscles and livers of aflatoxin-dosed birds. However, Rajesekher Reddy *et al.*(1982) could not detect the metabolites on the muscle or liver samples from the toxin-fed birds. The presence of toxic metabolities in the tissues may be dependent on the quantity and duration of feeding toxin, age of the birds, age of the birds, the route of administration of toxin and also the sensitivity of aflatoxin analysis.

Effect of aflatoxin on growth

Aflatoxin B_1 inhibits the nucleic acid synthesis, thus directly affects the transcription process in the protein synthesis. Toxin also inhibits the transnational process in protein synthesis (Chu, 1977). Experiments revealed that aflatoxin B1 inhibits synthesis of RNA and DNA human embryonic lung cells (Legator *et al.*, 1965). During the protein synthetic process, aflatoxin B_1 perhaps its metabolite (s) directly modifies the template rather than having a direct effect on enzyme systems.

The inhibition of protein synthesis immediately after the animal receives the toxin can be attributed primarily to inhibition at polyribosomal level and secondarily to impairment of transcription process, which to an inhibition of initiation of protein synthesis (Shank and Wogan, 1966). Aflatoxin effects the rough endoplasmic reticulum and cause dislocation of ribosomes. A direct inhibition on protein synthesis of elongation and/or termination stemp occurred at a low toxin does and at an early stage.

Dietary aflatoxin caused growth depression in broiler chicks. The lowest level of toxin dose, 0.25 ppm was considered to elicit effect on growth in broiler chicks Rajeskher Reddy *et al.*, 1982 and Nandakumar Reddy *et al.*,1982). Growth depressing effect of aflatoxin B_1 was demonstrated only after 2 weeks of feding aflatoxin at 1 ppm and above.

Feed consumption and feed efficiency

Aflatoxin B_1 and caused decreased feed consumption at 0.5 ppm and lowered feed efficiency (feed/gain in weight) at 1.25 ppm in broilers (Rajasekher Reddy *et al.*, 1982).

Effect of visceral organs

Liver and kidney were target organs to dietary aflatoxin. Aflatoxin B_1 caused increase in liver and kidney weights, at 0.5 and 0.75 ppm respectively. The liver fat was found to be increased at 0.75 ppm. Increased spleen weight was observed at 1.5 ppm (Rajasekher Reddy *et al.*, 1982).

Effect on livability

Aflatoxins can cause significant mortality in broilers at 1 ppm and above onwards. Apparently, higher levels of the toxin (at 1 ppm and above) caused graded mortality in a shorter period while smaller doses of toxin were found fatal over a longer period of feeding (Rajashekher Reddy *et al.*, 1982).

Effect on lipid metabolism

Aflatoxins altered lipid metabolism in broilers. A smallest dose of 0.625 ppm aflatoxin B_1 affected the transport of triglycerides, Phospholipids are cholesterol. Aflatoxin effected thiokinase enzyme thus alters lipid synthesis (Chu, 1977). A decrease in bile salts pancreatic lipase were also observed in chicken with experimental aflatoxicosis. Thus aflatoxin resulted in interference of lipid absorption and degradation (Smith and Hamilton, 1970). It is known that liver secretes triglycerides in conjugation with which plasma proteins into the bloodstream via the hepatic sinusoides which probably involves the endoplasmic reticulum (ER). The fatty livers subsequent to feeding aflatoxins in broilers might have occurred either due to the impairment of ER or decreased lipoprotein synthesis (Harris and Robinson, 1961).

Effect on carbohydrate metabolism

Aflatoxin caused the reduction of hepatic glycogen level. A significant decrease in UDP-glucose-glycogen transglucocylase, glycogeno-phosphorylase, phosphoglucomutase and glucose 6-phosphate activity was observed in chicken livers after injection of aflatoxin B_1 (Chu, 1977).

Effect on certain biochemical parameters

Aflatoxins in brolier caused increased carcass condemnation due to bruise formation on breath and thigh muscles. Increase in liver and muscle lysosomal activity was observed in broilers at 0.625 ppm aflatoxin. The lower serum protein levels associated with aflatoxicosis appear to be related to the observed increase in the liver lipid content. This condition was substantiated by the findings that an inhibition of protein synthesis was a key event in fatty metamorphosis of the liver (Harris and Robinson, 1961) and Robinson and Harris, 1961). Serum cholesterol and serum uric acid were found to decrease during aflatoxicosis (Nandakumar Reddy *et al.*,1984).

Effect on immunological organs

Immunological organs i.e. bursa of Fabricius and thymus were found to regress at 1.25 and 0.625 ppm aflatoxin B1 respectively (Rajesekher Reddy *et al.*, 1982 and Thaxton *et al.*,1974). Several explanations for the immuno suppression ability of aflatoxin were reviewed by Rajesekher Reddy (1980).

1. Aflatoxins inhibits synthesis of specific immunoglobulins through inhibition on RNA polymerase.
2. Enhanced degradation of antibodies due to the increased specific activity of Iysosomes by aflatoxin.
3. Inhibition of antigen process by aflatoxin through inhibitory effect on RE system.
4. Aflatoxin inhibits the integrity of specific immunological tissues like bursa and thymus, impairing the antibody production.

Aflatoxicosis was observed to cause an increase in bone fragility and interacts with vitamin D deficiency (Hamilton *et al.*, 1974). Absorption of mineral i.e. calcium and phosphorus were lowered incidental to aflatoxicosis (Huff *et al.*, 1977).

Increasing the protein content of diet gave essentially complete protection to broilers against 5 ppm of aflatoxin (Smith *et al.*,1971) and Subba Rao *et al.*, 1977). Lipid content of diet when increased from 2% to 16% reduced the mortality. Aureomycin significantly stimulated growth and feed conversion and decreased death rate when added at a level of 0.0055% to a diet containing aflatoxin (Smith *et al.*, 1971).

Effect on haematology

Erythrocyte count, PCV, HB levels in broilers were decreased by dietary aflatoxin at 1.5 ppm (Rajeshekher Reddy *et al.*,1983). As low as 0.25 ppm and 0.75 ppm of toxin affected the Hb and PCV respectively (Nankakumar Reddy *et al.*,1984). Erythrocyte counts were lowered at 0.625 ppm (Tung *et al.*,1975).

Bone marrow revealed a general hyperactivity of the marrow tissue including an elevated cytopoisis of the hererophilic elements. This was confirmed by chemical showing decreased fat and increased nucleic acid content of the bone marrow. A possible explanation for the anemia coupled with hyperactive bone marrow could be that aflatoxin caused the production of erythrocytes with an impaired integrity and thus a decreased half life. A dose-related hypertrophy of the spleen suggests this organ might be responsible for an enhanced removal of erythrocytes from circulation (Hamilton *et al.*,1971). Results obtained by Wyatt *et al.* (1973) suggested that aflatoxin can cause hemolytic anemia.

Age of the chicken influenced the effects of aflatoxin on haematological parameters, other birds appeared to be more resistant to the effects of aflatoxin (Lanza *et al.*, 1977).

Symptoms and gross pathology

Symptoms were not noticed in the birds at higher levels of aflatoxin (4 and 6 ppm). At 1 ppm and above level of aflatoxin. The birds were off-feed, dull, stunted. Atrophy of the breast muscle, wart-like growths on the legs and feet were common findings in birds on dietary aflatoxin (Rajashekher Reddy *et al.*,1983).

Dietary aflatoxin in broilers revealed pathognonomic lesions in liver and kidney (Rajeshekher Reddy *et al.*, 1983). The lives appeared mottled with round borders and pale yellow with pin point haemorrhages. The livers were pliable. Exposure of toxin for longer duration be due to the fibrosis of liver. Gall bladder distension was characteristic. Greyish necrotic changes on the surface of enlarged kidney were common. Splenomegaly and atrophy of bursa was also common feature of aflatoxin poisoning. Urate deposition was also evident in kidney.

Histopathology

Birds received aflatoxin at level of 1.5 ppm showed consistent lesion in various tissues like liver, kidney, bursa (Rajashekher Reddy *et al.*, 1983). Livers were highly congested. Mild fatty changes with fibroblastic proliferation in the portal areas were characteristic. Degenerative and necrotic foci was characterized by pyknosis and karyorrhexis.

Kidneys were congested, oedematous and with petechnical

haemorrhages. In bursa the lesions were lymphoid depletion in the follicles, proliferation of fibroblasts and interfollicular fibrosis.

REFERENCES

Archibald, R.M., H.J., Smith and J.D. Smith, 1962. Can, Vet J. 3 : 322-325.

Asplin, F.D. and R.B.A. Carnaghan. 1961. Vet. Rec. 73 : 1215-1219.

Chu. F.S. 1977. Appl. Microbiology Vol. 22 , pp. 83-147.

Gopal, T., S. Zaki, M. Narayanaswamy and S. Premalata. 1969. Ind. Vet. J. 46 : 348-49.

Hamilton, P.B., H.T. Tung and F.W. Cook 1971. Poult Sci. 50 : 1583 (Abstr.)

Hamilton, P.B., H.T. Tung , R.D.Wyatt and W.E. Donaldson, 1974. 53 : 871-874.

Harris, P.M. and D.S. Robinson. 1961. Biochem. J. 80 : 253.

Huff, W.E., J.A. Deorr and P.B. Hamilton. 1977. Poult Sci. 56 : 1724 (Abstr.)

Kratzer, F. H., D. Banely, M. Wiley and A.N. Booth. 1969. Proc. Soc. Exp. Biol. Med. 131 : 1281-84.

Kumar, J. B. and B.K. Gowdaveeranarayana. 1979. Indian Vet. J. 56 : 494-96

Lanza, G.K.W., K.W. Washburn and R.D. Wyatt. 1977. Poult Sci. 56 : 1352 (Abstr.)

Legator, M. S., S. M. Zuffante and A. R. Harp. 1965. Vet . Bull. 1966. 334 (Abstr.)

Nandakumar Reddy, D., P. V. Rao, V.R. Reddy and B. Yadagiri. 1984. Indian J. Anim. Sci., 54 : 68-73.

Phatnur, N. 1965. Vet Rec. 77 : 1028 (Abstr.)

Patterson, D.S.P. 1973. Food Cosmet. Toxicol. 11 : 287-294.

Rajashekher Reddy, A., V.R. Reddy, P.V. Rao and B. Yadagiri. 1982. Indian J. Anim. Sci. 52 : 405-10.

Rajashekher Reddy, A., V. R., Reddy, M. Mahender and P.V. Rao. 1983. Trop. Vet Anim, Sci Res. 1 : 159-164.

Rao, A. G., P. K. Dehuri, S. K. Chand, S. C. Mishra, P. K. Mishra and B. C. Das. 1985. Indian J. Poult. Sci. 20 : 240-244.

Rivelli Florentin, E., G. T., Coltier, U; L. Diener and M. D. Davis. 1969. Poult Sci. 48 : 1807.

Robinson, D. S. and P. M. Harris, 1961. Biochem. J. 80 : 361.

Shank, R. C and G. N. Wogan. 1966. In. Vet.Bulletin. 1967 : 2528 (Abstr.)

Smith, J. W. and P. B. Hamilton. 1970. Poult Sci. 49 : 207-213.

Smith, J. W, C. H., Hill and P. B. Hamilton. 1971. Poult Sci. 50 : 768-774.

Subbarao, I. V. R., K. S. Singh, R. K. Tripathi and B.S. Rao. 1977. Indian J. Poult Sci. 1 : 42-47.

Thaxton, J. P., H. T. Tung and P. B. Hamilton. 1974. Poult Sci. 53 : 721-25.

Tung, H. T., F. W., Cook. R. D. Wyatt and P.B. Hamilton. 1975. Poult. Sci. 54 : 1962-69.

Vanzyatreld, W. A., D. C., Kelley and Stanly M. Dennis. 1970. Poult. Sci. 49: 1350-1356.

Wyatt, R. D., H. T., Tung, F. W. Cook and P.B. Hamilton. 1973. Poult. Sci. : 2105 (Abstr.)

CHAPTER

12

MYCOTOXICOSIS OF LESS COMMON OCCURRENCE IN CHICKEN

A. Rajan,
Director, Centre of Excellence in Pathology, College of Veterinary & Animal Sciences, Mannuthy, Trichur

A large number of toxin metabolites are produced by fungal organisms and some of them have been identified as causative factors for diseases in man and animals. Among these toxins, aflatoxins are well known and extensive studies have been made on aflatoxicosis. Now aflatoxin has become synonymous to mycotoxins and unfortunately people forget about the involvement of other mycotoxins. There are a few other mycotoxins like ochratoxin, citrinin and trichotecenes which are important but has not been systematically looked for. Besides the toxicity of these fungal metabolites by themselves synergistic effects of these toxins when they occur simultaneously in natural situations have also to be borne in mind. It is becoming increasingly evident that a number of naturally-occurring mycotixins in addition to aflatoxin should be considered potentially dangerous to poultry.

Ochratoxicosis

Ochratoxin A (OA) is a nephrotoxic mycotoxin chiefly produced by *Pencillium viridicatum* and *Aspergillus ochraceous.* This toxin is well known since its association with porcine nephropathy was established by Larson (1928). The main toxin component is DA and later Ochratoxin B and were described.

Reviews on ochratoxicosis have documents (Styn. 1971 : Chu, 1974 and Carlton and Krogh, 1979). Recently Dwivedi and Burns (1986) made a review on ochratoxicosis in poultry. OA is a colourless crystalline compound with a molecular formula C20, H18 No 6. The toxin is heat stable and withstands autoclaving for 3 hours.

The first authenticated spontaneously-occurring ochratoxicosis in poultry is that of Hamilton *et al.* (1982) who investigated five independent outbreaks of ochratoxicosis involving large number of turkeys, ducks and chicken in the USA.

The broiler chicken had poor growth and layers had very low production and this was traced to consumption of contaminated corn. Viscent and Bottalico (1983) observed severe gastroenteritis in chicken fed mouldy bread. The bread was contaminated with *A. ochraceous* and contained 80 ppm of OA and 9.6 ppm of OB. Huff and Hamilton (1975) observed underpigmentation in broilers due to OA.

The minimum growth inhibiting level of the toxin was identified as 2 ppm. The LD_{50} by oral route was shown to be 166 ug (Chu and Chang, 1971). In broiler chicken the LD_{50} was identified as 2.14 ug/kg body weight (Pekham, 1975).

Huff *et al.* (1974) observed enlargement of the kidney, liver crop proventriculus and gizzard and regression of bursa. They also observed reduction in fibringogen and delayed clotting of blood and a clinical condition of 'bloody tight syndrome'. Hypochromic, microcytic anemia, inhibition of glycogenolysis and accumulation of glycogen in tissues and abnormal intramembraneous and endochondrial ossifications were also features of ochratoxicosis.

Huff and Doerr (1981) made a study on the synergistic effect of aflatoxin (2.5 ppm) and ochratoxin (2 ppm) in chicken and observed marked depression of growth, greater mortality and more severe kidney haemorrhagenthan in pure ochratoxicosis or aflatoxicosis.

According to Huff and Ruff (1982) a combination of OA and coccidiosis caused greater decrease in weight gain. Similarly a combination of OA (3 ppm) and tannic acid (1.5%) caused decreases in feather pigmentation and poor efficiency of feed utilization in broilers.

When OA was fed to 0 to 4 ppm to White Leghorn pullets from 14 weeks to one year there was delayed sexual maturity, decrease in egg production, weightgain and increase in feed intake with decrease in feed efficiency (Chaudhuri *et al.*, 1971).

Tohale (1983) observed reduced gain in weight and increased egg spots in Ochratoxicosis. In young chicken dehydration, dry firm gizzard, erosions in gizzard, haemorrghages in the proventriculous and catrrhal enteritis were reported. In broiler chicken enlarged pale kidney and visceral gout were observed. The bones became flexible and rubbery and in some cases brittle.

Campbell *et al.* (1983) fed broiler chicks OA (2 ppm) and aflatoxin (2.5 ppm) in the diet for 21 and 38 days from hatching. The effect of OA was marginal when given alone but when given in combination with aflatoxin was significant hypoprotenemia, lymphocytopaenia, heterophilia and reduced complement activity and decreased relative weight of bursa. The effect of OA on humoral and CMI was studied in detail by Dwivedi and Burns (1984). There was reduction in immunoglobulin and lymphoid organs showed reduced number of immunolobulin containing cells and suggested that OA is also an immunosuppressant. They gave OA at 2 ppm and 4 ppm levels to broiler chicken from the day of hatch. There was significant enlargement of the kidney, liver and proventriculus and the thymus of the bursa were reduced in size.

Hamilton *et al.*(1982) observed increased incidence of air sacculitis associated with ochratoxicosis and it was attributed to impaired immunoresponse. Immune response was depressed in a dose-related fashion in ochratoxicosis.

Histological changes described included tubular dilation, swelling of the epithelial lining, degeneration of the tubular basement membrane, hyaline casts in the tubules. The PCT was most severely affected. Thickening of the glomerular basement membrance as seen in mammals was not a feature (Dwivedi *et al.*,1984).

Dwivedi *et al.*(1984) observed glycogen storage in hepatocytes, focal areas of necrosis and haemorrhage, suppression of haematopoiesis, depletion of lymphoid elements from the spleen and bursa and pyknosis of ganglion cells in the brain.

Dwivedi *et al.*(1984) also described electron microscopic changes in ochratoxicosis in chicken. They observed abnormal mitochondria, increase in the size and number of mitochondrial dense gramules and cytoplasmic peroxicomes. They indicated that ring-shaped mitochondria were pathgnomomnic of ochratoxicosis The severity of changes was dose-dependent.

OA residues were detected in blood cells, plasma, muscle, liver, kidney and ovarian follicles by Juszkiewiez *et al.*(1982) and they focused the public health importance of the problem.

Fusariotoxicosis

T2 toxin (Trichotecenes) is a mycotoxin produced by several species of Fusarium. Wyatt *et al.*(1973) induced experimental toxicosis by feeding T2 toxin from 0, 1, 2, 4, and 16 ug/g of the toxin to broiler chicken. There are reduction in growth rate but the feed conversion was unaffected. The relative weight of the spleen was reduced and the weight of the pancreas was increased. At higher doses there was reduction in the weight of the bursa indicating the immunosuppressive effect of this toxin. There was no variation in the weight of the liver.

Oral lesions were characteristic of this toxin. Erosions and ulcers appeared first on the hard palate and along the margin of the tongue. Wyatt *et al.*(1973) observed neural disturbance characterised by loss of tighing effect of broiler chicken (the toxin was prepared from *F. poae*). Abnormal positioning of wings, hysterical seizures and falling on sides were also recorded. Joffe and Yagen (1977) fed pure T2 toxin from *F. sporotrichoides* to New Hampshire chicks and they observed necrotic enteritis, peticheae in proventriculus and haemorrhage in the liver and kidney.

Kubena *et al.*(1989) studied the combined effect of OA and T2. The effect were additive. They pointed out that in the natural situation this would be an important problem as both toxins will be present in the same feed.

Citrinin

This toxin was first isolated in 1931 *Pencillium citrium.* Like OA, this is also a nephrotoxin. Doerr and Cambell (1982) studied the combined effect of citrinin and OA in chicken (broilers). The broilers were given 0 and 400 ppm of citrinin and 0 and 2 ppm of OA for a period of 3 weeks. Body weight and feed conversion was reduced by the Ist week. Serum uric acid was elevated by OA but not by citrinin. Clagn *et al.* (1989) observed increased water consumption and excreate moisture and pointed out that these are important indicators of OA or citrinin toxicity. Osmoticdirresis and dehydration was due to failure of urine concentration by the kidney.

Summary

Ochratoxicosis, Fusariotoxicosis and citrinin toxicity and some of the mycotoxicosis which are important in addition to aflatoxicosis in chicken. OA and citrinin are nephrotoxins and T2 toxins causes mainly oral lesions. The lesions observed to these toxicosis have been described. The synergistic effects of these toxins in field situations are very significant and they may lead to great economic loss.

Suggestions for further reading

Choudhury, H. and Carlson, C.W.1973. Poult Sci. 52 : 1202

Doerr, J.A. and Campbell, M.C. 1982. Poult Sci. 61 : 1453.

Dwivedi, P. and Burns, R.P. 1984. Res. Vet. Sci. 36 (1) : 92

Dwivedi, P. Burns, R.P. and Maxwell, M.H. 1984. Res. Vet. Sci., 36 : 104.

Dwivedi, P. Burns, R.P. Res. Vet. Sci., 36 (1) : 117.

Dwivedi, P. and Burns, R.B., 1986. Poult Sci. 42 (1) : 32

Dwivedi, P. and Burns, R.B. 1986. Poult Sci. 42(1) : 48

Glahn *et al.* 1989. Poult Sci. 68(9) : 1041

Hamilton *et al.* 1982. Poult Sci. 61d : 1832.

Kubena *et al.* 1989. Poult Sci. 68.

Palti, J. 1978. Toxigenic Fusarium, their distribution and significance as a cause of disease in animals and man. Verlag Poul Parey, Berlin.

Prior *et al.*1976. Poult Sci. 56 : 786.

Wyatt *et al.* 1973. Poult Sci. 52 : 1853

Wyllie, T. and Morhorse, L.C. 1977. Mycotoxic fungi, Mycotoxins and Mycotoxicosis. Marcell Deckker, New York.

CHAPTER

13

MICOTOXIC NEPHROPATHY

Dr. S.M. Mohiuddin,
Associate Professor & Head, Department of Pathology, CVSs, Hyderbad.

Mycotoxic nephropathy is renal damage, caused by the ingestion of nephrotoxic fungal metabolites, produced by some toxinogenetic strains of the genus *Aspegillus* and *Pencillium* (*A. ocrraceus,*) *A. mellus, P. viridicatum, P. palitans),* which include sochratoxins, citrinins, oxalic acid and viridication toxins. These fungi are widely distributed in nature. They often invade cereals, maize, rice etc.

Ochrotoxin

Ochrotoxins include a group of strucuturally related secondly metabolites produced by seven species of *Aspergillus* and six species of *Pencillium* (Chu, 1974). *Aspergillus ochraceus.* from which the toxins acquired their name appear to be predominant ochortoxin producer (Chu, 1974).

Ochrotoxin A, which is the most toxic and most prevalent form is 7-carboxyl-5-chloro-8 hydroxyl-3,4-dihydro-3-R-methyl isocoumarin linked through an amide bond to L-B-phenylalanine (Vender Merwe *et al.*, 1965).

In poultry, limited research has been carried out on Ochotoxicosis. Huff *et al.* (1974) presented a general description of the disease in young broiler chickens and concluded that on the basis of acute mean lethal dose and minimal growth inhibitory concentration, Ochrotoxin-A is the most potent mycotixinyet studied in chickens. They also reportd that the most sensitive indicator of ochratoxicosis in young broiler chickens was enlarged kidneys. Microscopic evaluation of acute ochrotoxicosis of young White Leghorn cockerels (Doupnik *et al.*, 1970; Packham *et al.*,1971) revealed acute nephrosis, hepatic degeneration and suppression of hematopoiesis in descending order of frequency. On the other hand, histopathological study of ochratoxicosis in ducklings (Theron *et* *al.,*1965) revealed primarily hepatic degenerative changes in the matrix of the mitochondria and disorganization of the endoplasmic reticulum (ER) of hepatoctes. In laying hens ochratoxin at low concentrations delays sexual maturity, reduced egg production and hatchability.

Huff *et al.*(1975) studied the nephrotoxicity of ochratoxin. The effect of graded doses of ochratoxin A on the parameters measured are given in Table 1. The weight of the left kidney relative to the total body weight was increased by doses of 1 ug/g and above which agrees with the previous report (Huff *et al.,* 1974). At the highest dose, the relative kidney weight was more than doubled. The enlargement of the kidney could be the result of edema, a general increase of protoplasm, or an increase of a specific constituents.

The effect of dietary ochratoxin on the excretory function of the kidney was determined by measuring the rate of clearance of phenol red from the blood by the kidney. The rate of clearance was decreased significantly (P 0.05) at 4 ug and 8 ug/g. This alteration in the levels of blood constituents which are excreted by the kidney. The primary product of nitrogen catabolism in the chicken is uric acid (Sykes, 1971). The plasma uric acid levels were increased significantly, at dose levels of 4 and 8 ug/g. During kidney impairment an electrolyte imbalance is often seen. Serum potassium levels were decreased and the hypokalemia also was significant at 4 and 8 ug/g.

The most striking histopathological changes noticed in the kidneys during ochratoxicosis were swelling of the tubular epithelial cells, tubular dilation and protenacious material in the lumen. The proximal portion was more severely affected then the distal portion to the extent that some generalized necrosis of the epithelial cells of the proximal tubules was observed. Doupnik *et al.* (1970) and Reckham *et al* (1971) also observed similar changes due to ochratoxin in chicks.

According to Brown *et al.*(1985) the layer chicks treated with ochratoxin for 21 days showed normal glomerali, while the proximal tubular epithelial cells showed increased numbers of peroxisomes which were slightly larger as against the control birds. Mitochondria of some proximal tubular cells appeared narrow and tortuous. Ring-shaped mitochondria was present in both ochratoxin treated and control samples but were more common in the former. All the layer chicks treated with ochratoxin for 21 days had enlarged mitochondrial matrix granules in some cells. These enlarged granules had a hyaline electron lucent center and a dense margin. Proximal tubular cytoplasm also contained 0.8 to 1.2 um smooth round membrane-bound structures

Table1 : Effect of graded doses of dietary ochratoxin-A on parameters related to nephrotoxicity in broiler chicken

Parameter	Ochratoxin (ug/g)					
	0	0.5	1.0	2.0	4.0	8.0
Body weight (g)	415±65	413±40	405±60	335±20*	250±4*	107±25*
Kidney size (g100 g of body weight)	0.55±0.02	0.55±0.02	0.64±0.02*	0.66±0.02*	0.92±0.05*	1.17±0.05
Kidney dried weight (% of wet weight)	21.05±0.5	20.7±0.4	20.3±0.7	20.2±0.2	18.8±0.2*	15.2±0.4*
Plasma uric acid (mg/100 ml)	1.9±0.3	2.1±0.3	2.2±0.3	2.4±0.1	3.1±0.4*	3.7±0.2
Serum potassium (ug/litre)	5.5±0.2	5.5±0.1	5.3±0.2	5.2±0.1	4.8±0.2	4.6±0.1
Phenol red clearance (%)	63.8±0.8	59.7±1.7	66.0±1.7	63.4±1.5	4.3±1.7*	43.9±8.9*

interpreted as secondarynlsosomes. These structures were filled witha finely granular material and a few small dense granules. Some proximal tubular material and a few small dense granules. Some proximal tubular nuclei contained clear round vacuoles upto 1.5 um in diameter. Some vacuoles contained loose flocculent material and a central slightly electrondense granular round structure, but most were empty. Distal tubular and cortical collecting duct epithelium had no significant changes compared with those in control.

Citrinin

Citrinin, a fungal metabolite, was isolated and identified by Hetherington and Roistrick (1931). It is a nephrotoxin, which causes kidney degeneration and increased urine excretion. Ames *et al.* (1976) fed chicks diets containing 62.5, 12.5 250 and 500 ppm citrinin. All levels of the toxin caused, enlarged kidneys and there was a dose related increase in liver size, but body weight was decreased only at 500 ppm.

Roberts and Mora (1978) fed chcks, diets containing 33, 65, 130 and 260 citrinin. All levels of the toxin caused cellular infiltration in the liver, kidney and pancreas. Growth was depressed at 130 and 260 ppm citrinin.

Nelson *et al.* (1981) studied the citrining toxicity in growing chicks and concluded that the level of citrinin that would decrease growth in less than 330 ppm. Increased water excretion was noticed as one of the symptoms of citrinin toxicity.

Brown *et al.* (1985) studied the individual and combined effects of citrinin and ochratoxin-A on renal ultrastructure in layer chicks. The mechanism of action of citrinin in vivo has been established (Mehdi *et al.*, 1984), but it may also involve proximal tubular mitochondria, since the mitrochondrial shape changes are similar to those produced by ocharatoxin. The absence of inclusion in citrinin treated chicks suggested that mitochondria were not to the same degree as in citrinin toxicosis. This difference may be of assistance in the differential diagnosis of these two toxicosis. Increased numbers of the peroxisomal and other membrane-bound granules interpreted as secondary lysosomes were present in birds fed with citrinins for 24 days. Such increase may indicate an increase rate of organelle or cell turnover by autophage, since peroxisomes are increased around the sites of membrane injury and are enlarged with some toxin tubular injuries.

Oosporein

Oosporein is a toxin fungal digunone produced by Oosporal colorans (Kogl and Van Wessan, 1944), some chaetomium species (Cooke, 1970, 1973: Chu, 1974 : Cole *et al.*, 1974 : Lyoyed *et al.*, 1955) and numerous other mould species. The natural contamination of feed grains by chaetomium spp, and the toxicity of these grains to domestic and laboratory animals have been documented (Christensen *et al.*, 1988). The toxicity of purified oosporein has been studied only in poultry. The single oral dose LD50 values in broiler chicks were 5.77, 5.00 and 4.56 mg/kg body weight for oosporein acid, oosporein Na salt and oosporein K salt respectively (Manning and Wyatt, 1984).

Chicks and turkey poults fed oosporein had visceral and articular urate deposits, enlarged kidneys, proventicular erosion, green discolouration of the gizzard lining and elevated serum uric acid, levels (Pegram and Wyatt, 1981, 1982). These findings indicated that the kidneys are the major target organ for oosporein.

Brown *et al* (1987) indicates that oral oosporein K salt is nephrotoxic, and the effects the most severe in initial phoximal tubular (PT) segements. Renal ischmic damage in lower tubular segments (Yamamato *et al.*,1984) due to the renal effects of oosporein and probably not due to blood flow reductions.

Damage of initial and subsequent PT segments may be responsible for hyperuriemia and deposition of urates seen in acutely affected individuals. Under normal conditions, the serum uric acid of chicks is actively transported to PT ipithelial cells by a K-dependent anion pump in the basal membrane which is distinct from that of other organic anions (Zmuda, 1965). Tubular eipthaolial cells also synthesize uric acid from xanthene and guanine which diffuse passively into proximal tubules. Uric acid from both sources positively diffuses into tubular lumes down in an electro-chemical gradient. Upto 40% of secreted urate is resorbed by subsequent tubular segments in chicks (Shideman *et al.*,1981).Thus, selective destruction of initial tubular segements with sparing of subsequent segements as produced by oosporein could lead to decreased capacity for uric acid secretion and severe hyperurimia. Alternatively, decreasedrate of luminal flow in affected nephrons may inhibit uric acid diffusion at the luminal membrane and allow significant back leak into capillaries, as has been shown to occur in isolated snake oosporein directly inhibits proximal tubular uric acid pumps and prevents its excretion (Pegram and Wyatt,

1981). Mechanism, of visceral urate deposition, as seen during this trial are unexplained, but such deposition is an indication of terminal renal failure (Siller and Ostler, 1961).

SUMMARY

Mycotoxin induced disease is common in poultry and most outbreaks are characterized by hepatic disease, gastrointestinal losses or loss of body weight (Pegrum and Wyatt, 1981). Some mycotoxin also affect renal function and structures. In turkeys and ducks, aflatoxins induces nephrosis with period acid schiff positive granules in proximal tubular epithelial cells (Newberne *et al.*,1964 : Siller and Ostler, 1961 and Wannop, 1961). In broiler chicks, ochratoxin-A is a potent nephrotoxin causing proximal tubular nephrosis, thickened granular capillary basement membrane, abnormal mitochondrial shapes, and increased size and number of proximal tubular and lesions in medullary cones of poultry given a large oral dose (Mehdi and Carlton, 1981, 1984). Oosporein may be included in this group, since it produced hypeurimia and urate deposition leading to renal damage in chicks (Gibbs, 1929, Siller and Ostlter, 1961).

REFERENCES

Ames, D.D., R.D. Wyatt, H.L. Marks and K.W. Washburn. 1976. Effect of citrinin, a mycotoxin produced by pencillum citrinum on laying hens and young broiler chicks, Poult Sci, 55 : 1294-1301.

Brown, T.P., O.J. Fletcher, O. Osuna and R.D. Wyatt, 1987. Microscopic and ultra structural renal pathology of oosporein induced toxicosis in broiler chicks, Avi. Dis. **55** : 868-877.

Brown, T.P., R.O, Manning, O.J. Fletcher and R.D. Wyatt. 1985. The individual and combined effects of citrinin and ochratoxin-A on renal ultrastructure in layer chicks, Avi. Dis. **30**(1) : 191-198.

Chu, F.S. 1974. Studies on ochratoxin. Crit, Rev. Toxicol. **3** : 499-524.

Cole, R.J., J.W. Kirskey, H.G. Cutter and E.E. Davis. 1974. Toxic effects of oosporein from chaetomium trilaterate J. Agric, Food Chem. **22** : 517-520.

Christensen, C.M., G.H., Nelson. C.J. Mirocha and F. Bates. 1968. Toxicity of experimental animals of 943 isolates of fungi. Cancer Res. **28** : 2293-2298.

Cooke, J.C. 1973. Variation In isolates of chaetomium trilaterate. Mycolgia. **65** : 1212-1220.

Cooke, J.C. and R.P. Collins, 1970. Oosporein from chaetomium trilaterate, I. Loydia. **33** : 269.

Dantzler, W.H. 1982. Studies on non-mammalian nephrons. Kidney Int. **22**: 560-570.

Doupnik, B. and J.C. Peckham. 1970. Mycotoxicity of Aspergillus ochraceus to chicks. Appl. Microbiol. **19** : 594-597.

Dwivedi, P. and R.B. Burns. 1984. Ultrastructural study of the liver and kidney in ochratoxicons-A in young broiler chicks, Res. Vet. Sci. 104-116.

Dwivedi, P. and. R.B. Burns. 1984. Pathology of ochratoxicosis A in young broiler chicks. Res. Vet. Sci. **36** : 92-103.

Gibbs, O.S. 1929. The effects of drugs on the selection of uric acid in the facel. J. Pharmacol. Exp. **35** : 49-62.

Hetherington and Roistrick, 1931. Studies in the biochemistry of micro-organism part XIV. On the producion and chemical constituents of a new yellow colouring matter. Citrinin produced from glucose by pencillium citrinum. Tromphil Trans. Soc. (London) Series of B 220-269.

Huff, W.E., R.D., Wyatt, T.C. Tucker and P.B. Hamilton. 1974. Ochratoxicosis in the broiler chicken. Poult. Sci. **53** : 1585-1591.

Huff, W.E., R.D. Wyatt and D.B. Hamilton. 1975. Nephrotoxicity of dietary ochratoxin A in broiler chickens. Appl. Microbi. **30** (1) : 48-51.

Kogl, P. and G.C. Vavan Wessan. 1944. Utersuchungen ulser pilzferbstoffe, XIV. Uber Oosporein, den tarbstaffe van Oosporacolorans van Beyma. Rech. Trev. Chimo, Pays-Bas Belg **63** : 5-12.

Lloyd, G., A. Robertson, G.B. Sankey and W.B. Whalley. 1955. The chemistry of fungi part XXV. Oosporein, a metabolite of chaetomium aureum chivirs. J. Chem. Soc. 2163-2165.

Manning, R.O and R.D. Wyatt. 1984. Comparative toxicity of chaetonium contaminated corn and various chemical forms of oosporein in broiler chicks.poult. Sci. **63** : 251-259.

Mehdi, N.A.Q. and W.W. Carlton. 1981. Citrinin mycotoxicon in broiler chicken. Food Cosmet. Toxi. 19 : 723-733.

Mehdi, N.A.Q. W.W. Carlton, G.O. Boon and J. Tuite. 1984. Studies on the sequential development and pathogenesis of citrinin mycotoxicosis in turkeys and ducklings. Vet. Pathol. 21 : 216-223.

Nelson, J.N., A.E. Aslay, L.K. Kirby, Z.B. Johnson, G.C. Ballam, and M.M. Campbell. 1981. Citrinin toxicity in growth chicks. Poult Sci. **60** (9) : 2165-2166.

Newberne, P.M., W.W. Cartton and W.N. Wogan. 1964. Hapatomas in rats and hepatorenals injury in ducklings fed peanut meal or Aspergillus flavus extract. Patral. Vet. **1** : 105-132.

Pegrum, R.A. and R.D. Wyatt. 1981. Avian gout caused by oosporein, a mycotoxin produced by chaetomium trilaterate. Poult. Sci. **60** : 2420-2440.

Peckham, J. C. B. Doupnik and O. H. Jones. 1971. Acute toxicity of ochratoxins A and B in chicks. Appl. Microbi. **21** : 492-494.

Pegrum, R. A., Wyatt and T. C. Smith. 1982. Oosporeins toxicosis in the turkey poult. Avi. Dis. **26** : 47-59.

Roberts, W. T and F. C. Mora. 1978. Toxicity of pencillium citrinum AUA - 532. Contaminated corn and citrinin in broiler chicks, Poult Sci. **57** : 1221-1226.

Shideman, J. R., M. J., Zmuda and A. J. Quebbemann. 1981. The acute effects of furosemide, ultra crynic acid and the chlorothiazide on the renal tubular handling of uric acid in the chicken. J. Pharmacol. Exp. Thev. **216** : 441-446.

Siller, W. G. and D. C. Ostler. 1961. The histopathology of an entero-hepatro syndrome of turkey poults. Vet. Rec. 73 : 134-138.

Sykes, A. H. 1971. Formation and composition of urine. 233-278 pp. In O.J. Bell and B.M. Freeman (eds) **Physiology and Biochemistry of the Domestic Fowl.** Vol. I., Academic Press Inc., New York.

Theron, J. J., K. J. Vander Merwe, M. Leebenberg H. J. B. Joubert and W.Nel. 1965. Acute liver injury in ducklings and rats as a result of ochratoxin poisoning. J. Pathol. Bacteriol. **91** : 521-529.

Vander Merwe. K. J., P. S. Steyo and L. Fourie, 1965. Mycotoxins. Part. II. The consitution of ochratoxin A, B and C metabolites of Aspergillus ochraceous, J. Chem. Soc. 7083-7088.

Wannop, C. C. 1961. The histopathology of turkey 'X' disease in Great Britain. Avi. Dis. **5** : 371-381.

Yemamoto, K., D. R. Wilson and B. Reuben. 1984. Outer medullary circulatory defect in ischemic acute renal failure. Amer. J. Pathol. **116** : 253-261.

Zmuda, M. J. and A. J. Quebbemann. 1975. Localization of renal tubular uric acid transport defect in gouty chickens. Am. J. Physiol. **229** : 820-825.

CHAPTER 14

INFLUENCE OF MYCOTOXINS IN OUTBREAKS OF COCCIDIOSIS IN POULTRY

Dr. P. Padmavathi,
Associate Professor, Department of Parasitology, College of Veterinary Science, Rajendranagar, Hyderabad.

Avian coccidiosis is one of the major and the most prevalent diseases affecting poultry reared in modern intensive methods under almost every possible climatic condition. It is responsible for heavy economic losses in poultry industry. Studies to probe through the morphology life cycle, patholgenicity and immunity aspects of coccidia were undertaken since ages. Even under strict hygienic conditions and with the usage of coccidiostats in feed, outbreaks of coccidiosis are still surfacing.

Today, mycotoxin contamination feeds is a worldwide problem. Aflatoxin achieved notoriety during the early 1960s. Apparently, this toxin has been reported to cause heavy mortality in turkeys. the toxin damages the liver during the process of detoxification leading to decrease in the total serum protein, albumin concentration (Brown and Abrahm, 1965). The toxin also caused leucopenia and thymus involution. It is a hepato toxin, nephrotoxin and carcinogen (Elling *et al.*, 1975 : Huff *et al.*,1975). It has been proved that aflatoxins are immunosuppressive. They have a marked suppressive effect on the development of acquired immunity through its action on C.M.I. system (Pierce *et al.*,1980b). The ability of aflatoxin to depress protein synthesis may also have its possible effect on immunity development.

Tung and Hamilton (1973) in their experimental studies with dietary aflatoxin level of 1.25 ug/g or above found that it significantly lowered the concentration of plasma carotenoids and increased clotting time.

Michael *et al.* (1973) noticed the impairment of RES of chicken resulting in decrease in clearance rate during aflatoxicosis. They opined that chicken with aflatoxicosis may be more susceptible to infections because of their decreased ability to process the antigenic component.

Cell mediated immunity is the major defence mechanism in coccidiosis. Poultry health hazards elaborated by increased mortality, poor growth rates and loss of production are frequently associated with the presence of aflatoxin of feed. The levels of aflatoxin found in survey of poultry feed samples are frequently lower than the levels required to produce aflatoxicosis in the laboratory. In the same way, subclinical levels of coccidial infection in labs produce severe outbreaks outside the lab. So a serious though has to be given to whether these two i.e. aflatoxin and coccidia are interacting with each other to produce more pathogenicity. The study of this line has been undertaken by a few workers. Hamilton and Harris (1971) stated that the field outbreak of mycotoxicosis in farm animals are often complicated with certain infectious diseases as his field surveys for aflatoxins contamination in feed revealed levels too low in produce clinical aflatoxicosis.

The interaction between mycotoxin and bacteria has been documented by Smith *et al.* (1969) and Boonchuvit *et al.*, (1975). Their studies showed that, dietary aflatoxin increased the susceptibility of chicken to fowl typhoid and paratyphoid infections. Mycotoxin T-2 is said to produce a dose dependant depression on CMI response and has been reported that it synergistically interact with Salmonella to increase mortality rate.

As mycotoxins are immunosuppressors and especially impairs CMI response which is the major defensive mechanism against coccidiosis, the interaction of aflatoxin and coccidiosis may be an important factors in the coccidial outbreaks in poultry.

Studies pertaining to the influence of aflatoxin on the outbreak of coccidiosis are meagre. Edds *et al.*(1973) carried out experiments in chicks fed with aflatoxin B_1 diet at 0.2 ppm for 21 days and followed by infecting them with 1,00,000 *E. tenella* oocysts on 29th day. They concluded that the birds became more susceptible with heavy mortality rate.

+++ Exposed to *E. tenella* infection

@@@ Fed B_1 and exposed to *E. tenella*

^{000} Exposed to *E. tenella* and given coccidiostat

Fed B1, given coccidiostat

This indicates that factors associated with broiler resistance had evidently been reduced. The decrease of serum protein concentration associated with aflatoxicosis would be expected to influence the pathogenesis and morbidity of coccidia. Equally important observation made by the above authors was the trend to the appearance. The area appear less severely infected which is due to the fact that coccidiosis occurs on diets designed to promote proliferation of anaerobic bacteria in the intestine and it is a secondary complacity, the primary etiological agent being bacteria. These mycotoxins being antibiotic in nature will automatically reduce the severity of lesions in coccidiosis. So this atypical appearance of disease could confuse a definite diagnosis in the field. Additional care has to be taken to ensure that these two disease a causing agents (coccidia and mycotoxin) and not interacting to obscure a diagnosis.

Edds and Simpson (1976) studied the effect of prior exposure of birds to aflatoxins for 28 days, followed by 21 days recovery period, to caecal coccidiosis. They observed that the birds were more susceptible to caecal coccidiosis and had more persistent hepatic and caecal lesion than that produced by aflatoxin. These results support earlier (Edds, 1973) conclusions that factors associated with the resistance had been lowered by exposure to aflatoxin B_1. The interference with normal hepatic function probably decrease the synthesis of serum immunoglobulins which in turn adversely influenced the pathogenesis and morbidity rate. The increased susceptibility to caecal coccidiosis persists even thogh the chicks had regained normal appearance and weight gain.

Huff and Ruff (1982) conducted an experiment in day-old broiler chicks infected with *E. acervulina* or *E. tenella* and fed with Ochratoxin A in their feed at the level of 0.5, 1.0, 2.0, 4.0a and 8.0 mg/g and found a decrease in the severity of the lesion with *E. acervulina* and *E. tenella* species. This effect to limit the severity of coccidial lesion was opined that Ochratoxin acts as antibiotic. Ochratoxin-A on either of the species of coccidia produced a significant decrease in body weight gain, plasma cortico steroid levels and increase in feed conversion ratio than infected with either of the infections alone. This indicates that Ochratoxin-A and coccidial infection can interact to limit broiler performance.

The effect of Ochratoxin-A, *E. acervulina* infection and combination of both, on body weight, feed conversion and lesion score

Parameter	Coccidia	Ochratoxin ppm					
		0	0.5	1.0	2.0	4.0	8.0
Body wt/g	No	595±14	597±17	584±18	560+13	317±17	178±8
	Yes	506±14	509±12	481±14	442±13	263±13	263±0
Feed conversion rate	No	1.264±0.3	1.407±0.18	1.392±0.23	1.458±0.39	1.648±0.118	2.447±0.22
Feed consumed (weight gain)	Yes	1.311±0.23	1.573±0.64	1.55±0.7	1.728±0.29	1.86±0.91	2.574±0.37
Lesion score	No	0	0	0	0	0	0
Yes	4	4	3.9±0.01	3.95±0.15	3.05±0.05	3.44±0.27	

Ochratoxin-A and coccidiosis coupled with additive detrimental effect seen on such economically important parameters such as body weight, feed conversion rate and pigmentation of the potential economic ramification of the concurrent presence of these two diseases are apparent. They further observed that there is species related difference in the interaction between the two species of coccidia and Ochratoxin-A. Effect of Ochratoxin and coccidiosis on a specific parameters was related to themechanism by which the disease condition produces pathological changes.

E. acervulina apparently exerts its influence through a combination of malabsorption and metabolic imbalance whereas blood loss is the major contributing factor in physiological changes associated with *E. tenella* infection. Ochratoxin is primarily nephrotoxin. Thus the magnitude of nephrommegaly seen with Ochratoxin-A and coccidiosis in combination was equal to the effect of ochratoxin-A alone. With *E. acervulian* infection the effect seen on PCV and HB was the decrease directly attributable to the level of the ochratoxin-A. Conversely with *E. tenella* infection, the depression of PCV and HB levels was so severe that no further effect was seen from increasing levels of ochratoxin-A (Table).

The usual situation which will be met in field is the simultaneous presence of aflatoxin and coccidia. There are few reports on these lines.

Wyatt *et al.* (1975) observed a significantly higher mortality in birds, which were infected with *E. tenella* and given a diet containing 2.5 ug aflatoxing/g of feed than in birds with aflatoxicosis or coccidiosis alone.

Cumulative mortalities of birds infected with *E. tenella* during 4-6 P.I.

($) Birds fed with basal diet

(*) Birds fed with basal diet containing 2.5 ug afatoxin/g

(@) Birds fed with basal diet containing 2.5 ug aflatoxin/g + 99 ug Monesin/g

() Birds fed with basal diet containing 99 ug Monensin/g

This effect was seen even when a light coccidial infection was there. Light coccidial infecion alone proved to be not able to increase mortality or cause weight depression. In addition, the higher mortality in the combination began earlier. Both individually dietary aflatoxin

The effect of Ochratoxin-A, *E. tenlella* and *E. acervulina* on kidney weight, haematocrit and HB.

Parameter	Coccidia		Ochratoxin-A ug/g					
		0.0	0.5	1.0	2.0	4.0	8.0	
Kidney gms/100 g body wt.	*E. tenella*	No	0.44±0.01	0.49±0.02	0.5±0.01	0.78±0.04	1.14±0.06	1.07±0.07
		Yes	0.45±0.01	0.51±0.02	0.5±0.01	0.59±0.03	0.99±0.06	1.19±0.10
	E. acervulina	No	0.48±0.1	0.48±0.01	0.53±0.01	0.58±0.02	0.94±0.04	1.16±0.05
		Yes	0.41±0.01	0.43±0.01	0.48±0.01	0.58±0.02	0.88±0.04	1.16±0.11
Haematocrit	*E. tenella*	No	22.6±0.4	23.3±0.84	22.7±0.4	23.7±0.03	20.9±0.5	18.6±0.7
		Yes	16.5±0.70	17.0±0.50	16.9±0.6	17.7±0.7	16.1±0.9	18.2±1.4
	E. acervulina	No	23.8±0.4	23.3±0.6	22.6±0.4	22.8±0.4	20.8±0.6	16.8±0.7
		Yes	20.6±0.6	21.7±0.6	20.8±0.5	20.8±0.5	19.1±0.5	17.5±0.9
Haemoglobin		No	8.3±0.39	9.0±0.4	8.0±0.1	8.3±0.3	7.3±0.3	5.8±0.3
	E.tenella	Yes	5.3±0.3	5.5±0.3	5.3±0.3	5.3±0.6	5.3±0.3	5.7±0.9
		No.	7.6±0.1	8.2±0.2	8.3±0.1	8.0±0.2	6.7±0.2	5.0±0.2
	E.acervulian	Yes	7.7±0.2	7.7±0.1	7.6±0.1	7.5±0.3	6.5±0.3	5.4±0.6

and *E. tenella* signficantly reduced HB, PCV and plasma pigmentation and in combination resulted in more severe reduction in HB, PCV and plsma pigmentation. Profuse haemorrhages was observed and very little coagulated blood was haemorrhages was observed and very little coagulated blood was seen in caeca. This was attributed to aflatoxin which lowers the tissue integrity and interfere with normal clotting time by prolonging the clotting time. The prolonged clotting time may be due to reduction in fibrainogen and due to competition with Vit. 'K'. So these effects along with *E. tenella* increase the speed of haemorrhage in tur increases faecal score. The caeca was less distended giving a low lesion score.

This study indicates that subclinical coccidiosis may be accentuated by dietary aflatoxin. Ruff and Wyatt (1978) in their study on the influencd of dietary aflatoxin on the severity of Eimeria infection in broiler chicks reported that the interaction between thse two resulted in the increase in severity of the only certain manifestations of the infection with such as depressed weight gain, marked increase in mortality rate.

Effect of dietary aflatoxin (2.5 ug/g of diet) and *E. acervulina* on young female broilers

Aflatoxin	1 x 10^5 oocysts of *E. acervulina*	Mortality	Lesion score	Weight gain
-	-	0	0	218±8.0
+	-	0	0	167±6.0
+	+	10	3.8±0.1	60±11.0
-	+	0	4±0.1	134±9.0

Souther and Backer (1984) studied *A. acervulina* infection during aflatoxicosis in chicken. They reported that both coccidiosis and aflatoxicosis depressed weight gain, feed efficiency and plasma pigmentation. In combination with aflatoxin, the disease agent depressed these criterions to a greater extent when either one alone. The depression appears to be additive rather than synergistic.

Whitelock *et al.,* (1982) undertook the same type of study with turkey coccidia *E. adenoides.*They inferred that severity of coccidial infection was increased in combination with aflatoxin.

CONCLUSIONS

Mycotoxins are reported to influence the outbreaks of Mareks, Salmonellosis and coccidiosis. The effect is brought about by suppressing CMI response. Mycotoxins are also responsible to increase the susceptibility to the above disease by interfering in the intermediary metabolism.

REFERENCES

Bomchurit, B., Hamilton, P.B. and Burmeister, H.R. 1975. Poultry Sci. 54 : 1693-1696.

Brown, J.M.M. and Abrams L. 1965. Onderstepoort J. Vety. Res. 32 : 119-145.

Edds, G.T., Nair, K.P.C. and Simpson, C.F. 1973. Am. J. Vety. Res. 34 : 819-26.

Edds, G.T. and Simpson, C.F. 1976. Am, J. Vety, Res. 37: 65-68.

Elling, F., Hald, B., Jacobrco, C. and Krogh, V.P. 1975. Acta Path, Microbiol. Scand Sec, A., 83 : 739-741.

Hamilton, P. B. and Harris, 1971. Poult Sci., 50 : 906-908.

Huff W. E. and Ruff, M. D. 1982. Poult Sci. 61 : 685-692.

Huff., W.E., Wyatt, R. D. and Hamilton, P.B. 1975. Appl. Micro. 30 : 48-51.

Michael, G. Y., Thaxton, P. and Hamilton, P.B. 1973. Poult Sci., 52 : 1206.

Pierce, A. C., Richard, J. L. and Thurston, J.R. 1980b. In Medical Mycology (H.J.Preusser, ed.) pp. 301-309, Fischer, Stuttgart.

Ruff, M. D. and Wyatt, R. D. 1978. Avian dis. 22 : 471-480.

Smith, J. W., W. R. Prince and Hamilton. P.B. 1969. Applied Micriobiol. 946-947.

Southern, G. L. and Baker, D. H. 1984. Nutrition Reports International, 29 : 35-44.

Tung, H. T. and Hamilton, P. B. 1973. Poult Sci. 52 : 80-83.

Whitlock, D. R., Wyatt, R. D. and Anderson, W. I. 1982. Poult Sci., 61 : 1293-97.

Wyatt, R. D. and M. D. and Page, R. G. 1975. Avian Dis., 19 : 730-740.

CHAPTER

15 TOXIC SYNERGISM BETWEEN AFLATOXIN AND OCHRATOXIN IN POULTRY

Dr. P. Ramo Rao,
Professor & Univ. Head, College of Veterinary Science, Tirupati.

A renaissance in mycotoxin research developed as a sequel to cocurrent outbreaks of disease in poultry and fish during 1960 in diverse geographical locations. The important report of severe losses in turkey poults was by Blount (1961) in England and named as Turkey X disease since etiology of the disease was not known. Later the responsible metabolites of the fungus was identified and designated as "Aflatoxin" (Sargeant *et al.*,1961). Ochratoxins were discovered while screening a large number of fungal cultures in the laboratory for toxicity by South African workers. Scott (1965) attributed for toxicity of a strain *A. ochraceus* Wilbelm to Ochratoxin a. causing nephrotoxicity associated with consumption of mouldy barley in Ireland.

The animal industry, particularly poultry is vulnerable in view of the use of high energy feeds which are incidentally preferred substrates for some toxic fungi. This is of much more importance in tropical coutries like India, wherein the climatic conditions, unseasonal floods, humidity and post harvest facilities are congenial for the growth of these toxigenic fungi on various feed ingredients like maize, groundnut cake, wheat bran etc. It is possible but not probable that conditions restricted growth to only one fungus. So when one mycotoxins in a commodity, the probability of presence of other mycotoxins is high. The synergistic or antigonostic effects of these mycotoxins is very imporant as these can alter clinical signs and lesions that differ from the individual effects. This fact makes the emphasizes the need to characterise mycotoxin interactions fully so that these can be recognized in the field.

Although the toxic effects of aflatoxin and ochratoxin in poultry is widely studied the literature on the synergisitc effects of these mycotoxins is scanty. An attempt is made in this paper to bring out the toxic synergism of aflatoxin and ochratoxin visa-vis the effects of the individual toxins in poultry.

Growth rate

Aflatoxin: A significant reduction in growth rate was reported in birds fed with 1.5 ppm aflatoxins (Carnaghan *et al.*, 1966 : Smith and Hamilton, 1970; Dalvi and McGowan, 1984 and Chattopadhya *et al.*, 1985).

Ochratoxin: A growth retardation in broilers by ochratoxin at doses of 1 ppm was reported by Huff *et al.*(1974), Campbell (1983) and Dwivedi and Burns (1984). The protein metabolizing systems are impaired.

Combined effect : A significant (PL 0.05) decrease in body weight of birds given aflatoxin and ochratoxin simultaneously at the synergisitic toxicity. The effect of the combination was far greater than the sum of the individual toxicity of these mycotoxins. The individual mycotoxins decreased body weight at 3 weeks of age by 12% each, while the combination of these mycotoxins decreased body weight of 40%.

Feed consumption and conversion: A dose dependent effect on feed consumption and conversion was reported with aflatoxin by Smith *et al.*(1984) and Chattapadhyaya *et al.*(1985) while no effect on feed conversion was noticed in ochratoxin treatment and combined interaction (Huff and Doerr, 1981).

Mortality: Mortality rate was increased in birds as a result of synergistic effect than that given alone of either toxin (Huff and Doerr, 1981).

Symptoms

Retarded growth, jaundice, coagulopathy in the form of excessive bleeding and dehydration of combs and shanks were the prominent symptoms in aflatoxcicosis (Chattopadyaya *et al.*,1985) while dullness, huddling, decreased appetite, weakness and diarrhoea in birds given 2-4 ppm of ochratoxin (Dwivedi and Burns, 1984). Nervous symptoms such as mild tonic convulsions and loss of righting reflex was reported in acute ochratoxicosis by Huff *et al.*, (1974).

Symptoms in synergistic effect of these two toxins was not documented.

Haematology

Anaemia characterised by a significant decrease in HB level and

PCV was a feature of individual toxicosis (Tung *et al.*, 1975 : Huff *et al.*,1988) and synergistic effect (Campbell *et al.*, 1983). In aflatoxicosis, blood clotting time was increased (Chattapodhyaya *et al.*,1985).

Liver lipids

Aflatoxin significant (PL 0.05) increased the lipid content of liver but ochratoxin did not alter. However, when both mycotoxins were fed, there was no altercation in lipid content (Huff and Doerr, 1981). Ochratoxin A seems to spare the lipid accumulation effect of aflatoxin in the liver.

Relative weight of organs

A significant increase (PL 0.05) in the relative weight of liver, kidney, spleen and proventriculus was reported in aflatoxicosis (Carnaghan, 1966 : Huff and Doerr, 1981) Whereas there was significant decrease in weight of bursa fabricius (Campbell *et. al.*,1983).

In ochratoxicosis, Dwivedi and Burns (1984 reported an increase in the weight of liver proventriculus and marked increase in the size of kidneys 1½ to 2 times the normal. Affinity of ochratoxin to gestrointestinal tract as seen by the enlargement of crop, proventriculus and gizzard was reported (Huff *et al.*, 1984).

No synergistic effect on the relative weight of liver was observed by Huff and Doerr (1981). However, they observed a significant increase (P/0.05) in the relative weight of kidney due to synergistic effect.

Gross pathology

Aflatoxin: The liver was the target organ which ws enlarged, soft, pale yellow with patechiae (Carnaghan *et al.*, 1966). Mottled livers with borders somewhat firm was reported by Vanzytveld *et al.* (1970).

Other changes noticed were pale and enlarged kidneys, pale and yellow spleen, patechiae over the heart and atrophy of Bursa (Chattopadhyaya *et al.*, 1983).

Ochratoxin: Liver was pale, enlarged and friable with pale and less viscous bile (Huff *et al.*, 1974) and Dwivedi and Burns, 1984).

Kidneys were pale and enlarged with distinct lobes beyond normal skeletal limits. Spleen and heart was increased in sizes. Cogestion and occasional haemorrhages in thymus, bursa was recorded. Slooughing of superficial layers of crop, proventriculus and gizzard was reported (Huff *et al.*, 1974).

Synergistic effect

Kidneys were significantly enlarged in birds given aflatoxin and ochratoxin together indicating that the synergisitc effect is mostly on the kidney (Huff and Doerr, 1981).

Microscopic lesions

Aflatoxin: Sequential changes in the liver of chicks fed with 1.5 ppm of aflatoxin was reported by Carnaghan (1966), Vanzytveld *et al.,* (1970) and Chattapadyaya *et al.* (1985). The main features were swelling of hepatocytes, fatty changes, bileduct hyperplasia, progressive fibrosis, regenerated eipithelial cells and haemorrhages.

Tubular degenerative changes were reported in the kidney (Vanzytveld *et al.*, 1970) Deplection of lymphoid cells with haemorrhages in the bursa fabricius.

Ochratoxin: In liver mild degeneratived changes, necrossis and peripotal fibrosis with inflammatory reaction was reported (Dwivedi and Burns, 1984 : Subramaniam and Govindaswamy, 1985).

A detailed study of changes in kidney was reported by Dwivedi and Burns (1984). The changes were enlargement of proximal and few distal converted tubules with homogeneous hyaline globules in the limen and nodular infiltration of lymphoid cells.

Subramaniam *et al.,*(1986) reported tubular nehprosis, fatty changes of distal convuluted tubules and glomerular epithelium and fragmentation of glomerular capillaries.

Depletion of lymphoid features and haemorrhage was a feature in lymphoid organs such as spleen, bursa fabricius and thymus.

Combined effects: Aflatoxin is primarily a hepatotoxin while ochratoxin, a nephrotoxin produces changes in liver and kidney respectively when given individually. But, the most sensitive organ to the combined effect of these two mycotoxins is the kidney. Synergistically pathological changes were more pronounced in the kidney.

Residual effects; There is no evidence to suggest that aflatoxin is stored in any tissue (Gildblatt, 1969). It would appear from the evidence now available that only food products from farm animals fed with ration containing aflatoxin, which might constitute a hazard to human health would be milk and milk products.

Micco *et al.*(1988) studied the residual effect of combined feeding of aflatoxin and ochratoxin and reported a higher content of ochratoxin in the liver of broilers (40 versus 5.0 ug/kg) and to lesser extent in kidney and skin and of aflatoxin in liver and kidney (0.15 versus 0.02 ug/kg and 0.40 versus 0.05 ug/kg, respecvively indicating a synergistic effect of ochratoxin and alfatoxin B, particularly in broilers.

CONCLUSION

Aflatoxin is primarily a hepatotoxin and a presumptive diagnosis can be made based on enlarged, firable and pale livers observed in chicks suspected to have consumed aflatoxin contaminated feed. Likewise ochratoxin, which is 3 times more toxin than aflatoxin in broiler chicks is primarily a nephrotoxin. In ochratoxicosis, enlargement of kidney is marked with discolouration. This distinction between aflatoxin and ochratoxin is useful in the field diagnosis.

The most sensitive organ to the synergisitc effect of these two mycotoxins is the kidney. Involvement of the kidney and reduced liver lipid accumulation would be viewed as symptoms atypical of aflatoxicosis. A diagnostician encountering such manifesation would probably discount the possibility of aflatoxin contamination further more, analysis for ochratoxin alone more not be expected to indicate levels sufficient to produce the symptoms observed.

It is apparent from the information that synergistic effect exists between aflatoxin and ochratoxin enhancing that toxicity. The symptoms patterns is so altered, the preliminary diagnosis during multiple mycotoxicosis is confusing. Further, studies on the synergism among these mycotoxins is required to provide valuable diagnostic information and a better understanding of the importance of mycotoxins to the livestock industry.

REFERENCES

Blount, W.P.C. 1961. "Turkey 'X' diseases - Turkeys - J. Brit. Turkey Federation 9(2) 52-77. Aflatoxin 1969. Ed. by Gold blatt - LA. pp.l.)

Campbell, M.L. Jr., May, J.D. Huff, W.E. and J.E. Dotrr. 1983. Evaluation of immunity of young broiler chicken during simultaneous administration of aflatoxin, ochratoxin. Poult Sci., 62 : 2138-2144.

Carnaghan, R.B.A., Lewis, G., Petterson, D.S.P. and R. Allcroft. 1966 Biochemical and hiological aspects of groundnut poisoning in chicken. Path, Vet. 3 : 601-615

Chattopadyaya, S.K., Taskar, P.K. Schaebe, O., Das, Y.T. and Brown, H.D. 1985. Clinical and biochemical effects of aflatoxin in feed ration of chicks. Cancer Bichem. Biophys. 8 : 67-75.

Dalwi, R.R. and Brown, C.M.C. 1984. Experimental induction of chronic aflatoxicosis of chickens by purified aflatoxin B_1 and its reversal by activated charcoal phenobutosol and reduced glutathione, Pullt Sci., 63 : 485-491.

Dwivedi, P. and Burns, R.B. 1984. Pathology of Ochratoxicosis in young broiler chickens. Res. in Vet. Sci., 36 : 92-103.

Goldblatt, L.A. 1969. Aflatoxin : Scientific background, control and implications. New York Academic Press, pp. 261.

Huff, W. E., Wyatt, R. D., Tucker, T. L. and Hamilton, P.B. 1974. Ochratoxicosis in the broiler chicken. Poult Sci., 53 : 1585-1591.

Huff, W. E. and Doerr, J. A. 1981. Synergism between aflatoxin and ochratoxin A in broiler chicken. Poult. Sci., 60 : 550-555.

Huff, W. E., Kubena, L. F. Harney, R. B. and Doerr, J. A., 1988. Mycotoxin interactions in poultry and swine. J. Anim. Sci., 66 ; 2351-2355.

Micco, C., Miraglia, M., Benulli, L., Oncer, R., Loppilo, A. and Montovan, A. 1988. Long term administration of low doses of mycotoxin in poultry. Residues of ochratoxin A and aflatoxin in broilers and laying hens after combined administration of ochratoxin A and aflatoxin. Food additives and containments. 5(3) ; 309-314 (Rev. of Med. of Vet. Mycol. (1988) 23 (3) : Abst. 1965.

Sargeant, K., Sheriden, A. O., Kelly, J. and Carnaghan, R. B. A. 1961. Toxicity associated with certain samples of groundnuts. Nature 192 : 1096-1097.

Scott, D. B. 1965. Mycopathol. Mycol. Appl., 25 : 213.

Smith, J. W. and Hamilton, P.B. 1970. Aflatoxin in the broiler chicken. Poult. Sci., 49 : 207-215.

Subramanian, S. and Govindaswamy, S. 1985. A ochraceous toxicity on carbohydrate metabolism in chicken. Current Science India 54 : (17) 860-862. Vet. Bull (1986) 56 (5) : Abst. 2965.

Tung, H.J., Cook, F.W., Wyatt, R.D. and Hamilton, P.B. 1975. The anemia caused by aflatoxin. Poult. Sci., 54 : 1962.

Venzytveld, W.M.A., Donald, C. Kulley and Standey, M. Dawins. 1970. Aflatoxicosis: The presence of aflatoxin and their metabolites in livers and skeletal muslces of chicken. Poult Sci. 49 : 1350-56.

CHAPTER

16

MOLECULAR ASPECTS OF AFLATOXIN B_1 IN MUTAGENICITY, TERATOGENICITY AND CARCINOGENICITY

Dr. A. Janardhan,
Associate Professor & Head Department of Pharmacology & Toxicology, CVS, Rajendranagar.

Through their use of sorcery and medicine, ancient civilizations already had some idea of the toxicity of fungi. With grain storage becoming a more common reality and the contant threat of spoilage due to adverse weather conditions or faulty storage facilities, the threat of mycotoxins present in the diets of animals of humans is obvious.

Of all the toxin-producing fungi other than ergot, *Aspergillus flavus* has received the most intense study due to its discovery in a common food stuff and its spectacular initial effect upon the birds of England.

The aflatoxins are the most potent of the currently recognised mycotoxins. Concentrations as low as 50 ppb aflatoxin B_1 can cause hepatic damage in laboratory animals. In swine, aflatoxin B_1 dietary levels of 0.5 ppm result in growth retardation and abortions. Feed levels of 1 to 2 ppm or more are capable of causing acute death in most species of livestock.

Chemistry

Aflatoxins are polycylic, unsaturated compounds consisting of a coumarin nucleus flanked by an apparently highly reactive bifuran system on one side and either a pentenene (B toxins) or a 6-membered lactone (G series) on the other. These toxins are relatively heat-resistant and not soluble in water. They are extractable from feed stuffs by a number of organic solvents. The addition of fungicidal dyes (eg-gentian violet) may help to prevent the production of aflatoxins in feeds, but will not destroy the aflatoxins already present.

Toxicodynamic considerations

Aflatoxins are absorbed from the intestinal tract and bound to serum albumin (Bassir and Babubunmi, 1973). Liver cells take up aflatoxin from blood. The rate of uptake depends on aflatoxin structure and the species. Within the hepatocyte, aflatoxins may exert direct effects on sex steroid binding sites on the endoplasmic reticulum. In the microsomes, aflatoxins are metabolised to various forms, one or more of the forms may be major active forms in some species (Ciegler, 1975). The toxins appear in the milk of lactating cattle (Allcroft and Robberts, 1968). Aflatoxins do not accumulate preferentially in any specific tissue but are excreted through the kidney as nonfluorescent water-soluble sulflates and glucuronides.

Mechanism of action

A number of biochemical changes occur which are secondary to the cytotoxic actions of aflatoxins. These changes include increases in SGOT, SGPT, blood alkaline phosphatase and bilurubin. There are decreases in serum protein and urea (Gumbmann and Williams 1969; John and Miller, 1969: Buck *et al.*, 1973; Hayes and Hannan, 1973). There is also an immuno-suppressie effect of aflatoxin (Pier, 1973; Thurston *et al.*, 1974). Aflatoxin has a major effect on cell mediaed immune (CMI) response. It produces thymic aplasia, reduces delayed cutaneous hyper-sensitivity (DCM) and graft verses host (GVH) responses and diminishes the phagocytic response of macrophages. Aflatoxin also diminishes the phagocytic response of macrophages. Aflatoxin also impairs complement (C_4) activity. Humoral effect of aflatoxin and include reduction of I_gG and I_gA but not impaired in most systems.

1.	Protein synthesis	Inhibitio (binds DNA, RNA, blocks transcription)
2.	Lymphoid tissue	Thymic aplasia
3.	Cell mediated immunity effects	DCH supressed responses GVH suppressed responses
4.	Phygocytes	Phagocytosis by Macro-phages reduced
5.	Humoral effects:	
	Complements	C4 reduced
	Antibody	Generally unchanged titer
	Immunoglobulin	IgG IgA reduction

In rat hepatocytes the first ultrastructural change elicited by aflatoxin B1 is a change in the nucleolar structure (Detroy *et al.*, 1971). The nuclelar damage is constant with observations that aflatoxin binds with nuclear DNA, which prevents DNA from acting as a templete (Buck *et al.*,1973) ; Wagan, 1974 and (1975). Therefore, nucleic acid polymerases cannot function leading to a decrease in ribosomal protein synthesis.

Subsequent ultrastructural changes include a decrease in smooth endoplasmic reticulum, loss of glycogen and mitochondrial degeneration (Detroy *et al.*,1971). These changes are consistent conseuqences are (1) aflatoxin B_1 inhibits, the electron transport system of mitochondria by acting between cytochromes B and C in vitro (Doherty and Campbell, 1972), (2) aflatoxin B_2 a major metabolite of B_1 covalently binds to rat live microsomal protein in vitro (Gurtoo and Dahms, 1974). Such actions could give rise to cell death.

Aflatoxins are thought to be metabolized to highly reactive *epoxides* and *phenolates* (the furan system of aflatoxin is involved here) that can bind and interfere with nucleic acids and proteins (Ciegler, 1975). Thus not only is the parent molecule capable of binding of cellular structures, but are also its metabolites *epoxides* and *phenolates.*

The expoides and phenolates are normally conjugated with glutathione that serves to protect vital macromolecules form these toxin intermediates. Hepatic necrosis is thought to result when glutathione reserves have been drastically depleted by conjugation with toxin intermediates so that the toxin intermediates are free to bind covalently to vital cellular macromolecules. Therefore it would be very interesting to find out, the reason why a high protein diet protects rats against aflatoxin. May be the protection is due to the presence of cystine (200 mg/kg b-w). While the glutathione depleting agent diethyl meleate (0.6 ml/kg) enhances the hepatotoxicity.

The big problem in studying the mechanism of action of aflatoxins is in determining which biochemical interactions are closely related to carcinogenesis, mutagenesis and teratogenesis on the one hand and hepatic degeneration and necrosis on the other. It appears that the mechanism overlap considerably.

Acute toxicity, genotoxicity and carcinogenicity of AFB_1 depend on the its metabolic activation. These adverse effects can be attributed to its capability of covalently binding to cellular target relevant for mutagenesis and carcinogenesis.

AB1 induces mutations in bacteria, algae and fungi, in insects and in various mammalian cell systems, including human cells. The mutagenicity of AFB_1 almost invariably depends on metabolism by the microsomal mixed function monoxgenase system. In absence of microsomal metabolism AFB_1 is a very weak mutagen, but in the presence of near UV light AFB_1 can be photocativated and induces mutations in bacteria.

Investigations have established that activated aflatoxins convalently bind to macro-molecular cell constituents i.e., DNA, RNA and protein (this binding occurs in vitro as well as in vivo).

Aflatoxin B is one of the most potent carcinogens inducing mainly liver cancer in the many experimental animals including primates. Direct evidence that AFB_1 is carcinogen for humans is lacking. However, the daily intake of AFB1 calculated from the dissemination of primary liver cancer among humans in Kenya, Switzerland, Mozambique and Thailand. This strongly suggests that AFB1 could be the causative agent of human liver cancer in those areas.

Aflatoxin may be considered as a biosynthetic inhibitor, large doses casuing total inhibition and lower doses progressively affecting different system. The successive stages in biological activity of aflatoxin on the liver cell can be tabulated as follows, each step being a consequence of the previous one:

1. Interaction with DNA and inhibtion of polymerases responsible for DNA and RNA synthesis
2. Suppression of DNA synthesis
3. Reduction of RNA synthesis and inhibiton m-RNA
4. Reduction in protein biosynthesis

DNA molecules present in the impaired cell no longer act as suitable models for their duplication. This failure of DNA duplication is analogous with the action of *actinomyesin* the structures of the two molecules have some features in common). Actinomyesin inserts itself into the double helix of DNA at a site containing *guinine (adenine* and *thymine* remain unchanged).

Aflatoxins may also affect the biosynthesis of RNA preventing the transcription of DNA by RNA polymerase. The activity of cytoplasmic RNA is totally inhibated whereas nuclear RNA is less so.

Phenobarbital, a microsomal stimulant, induces enzymes involved in hydroxylation reaction in the liver leading to the metabolism of aflatoxin in non-carcinogenic products.

The mutagenic activity of aflatoxin has been demonstrated by a variety of different procedures. the following systems have been used to establish this mutagenic activity. Microorganisms, cytogenetic effects in cultured mammalian cells, and dominent lethal tests in mice. Aflatoxin is now known to produce all forms of genetic damage i.e., carcinogenicity, teratogenicity and mutagenicity.

Since the work of Hale and Warkany on birth defects produced by variation in dietary Vit. A, it has been recognised that the developing fetus is particularly vulnerable to adverse influences in its environment. Studies of malformations at birth remained largely in the hands of peadiatricians who quickly established the connection between rubella infection in early pregnancy and the birth of severely affected infants. Dramatic increases in the incidence of phocomelia in new-born infants in Germany, the UK, Japan and other countries were traced to the use of an apparently non-toxic sedative thalidomide by pregnant women. It was through this tragic event of 1962, toxicologists were brought face to face with the devastating possibility of the chemically-induced developmental abnormalities.

A consideration of the role of the placenta in the developmental toxicology suggests that four aspects of placental function require consideration. These are:

1. The effects of toxic chemicals on the imporant reproductive function of the placenta
2. The interactions of the toxic chemicals with the products of placental metabolism in terms of effects on maternal and fetal organisms.
3. The capacity of the placenta to act as a regulator of the transfer of toxic chemicals from the maternal to fetal circulation
4. The capacity of placental enzyme systems to catalyse the generation of reactive toxic intermediates.

REFERENCES

Bassior, O. and Bababunmi, E.A. 1973. The binding of aflatoxin B with serum albumin. *Biochem. Pharmacol.* **22** : 132.

Ciegler, A. 1975. Mycotoxins : Occurrence, chemistry, biological activity. Loydia **38** : 21

Allcroft, R. and Roberts, B.A. 1968. Toxic groundnut meal : The relatioship between aflatoxin B intake by cows and excretion of aflatoxin M in milk. *Vet. Rec.* **82** : 116.

Gumbmann, M.R. and Williams, S.N. 1969. Biochemical effects of aflatoxin in pigs. *Toxical . Appl Pharmacol.* **15** : 393.

Joh, D.W. and Miller, L. L. 1969. Effect of aflatoxin B_1 in net synthesis of albumin fibrinogen and a-acid glycoprotein by the isolated perfused rat liver. *Biochem. Pharmacol.* **18** : 1135.

Buck, W.B., Osweiler, G.D. and Van Gelder, G.A. 1973. Clinical and diagnostic veterinary toxicology. *Dubugug,* Iown : Kendall/Hunt.

Hayes, A.W. and Hannan, C.J. 1973. Effect of rubratoxin and aflatoxin and oxygen consumption of krebs cycle intermediates. *Toxicol. Appl. Pharmacol.* **25** : 30.

Pier, A.C. 1973. Effects of aflatoxin on immunity. *J. Am. Vet. Med. Assoc. 163* : 1268.

Thurston, J. R. Deyoe, B. L., Bactz, A. L., Richard, J. L. and Booth, G. D. 1974. Effect of aflatoxin on serum proteins. Complement activity and antibody response to Brucella abortus in guinea pigs. *Am. J. Vet. Res.,* **35 :** 1097.

Wagan, G. N. 1974. Biochemical effects of aflatoxins. *Isr. J. Med. Sci.,* **10** : 441/

Wagan, G. N. 1975. Mycotoxins, *Annu, Rev. Pharmacol.* **15** : 437.

Detroy, R. W., Lillehoj, E. B. and Ciegler, A. 1971. Aflatoxin and related compounds. In :**S. Ciegler, S. kadis and S. J-Ajil** eds. *Microbial toxins. Vol.* 6 , N.Y. Academic Press.

Doherty, W. P. and Campbell, T. C. 1972. Inhibition of rat liver mitochondria electron transport flow by aflatoxin B_1. *Res. Commun. Chem. Pathol. Phrarmacol.* **3 :** 601

Gurtoo, H. L. and Dahms, R. 1974. On the nature of the blinding of aflatoxin B_{2a} to rat hepatic microsomes. *Res. Commun. Chem. Pathol. Pharmacol.* **9:** : 107.

Reid, W.D., Krishna, G. Gillette, J. R. and Brodie, B.B. 1973. Biochemical mechanism of hepatic necrosis induced by aromatic hydrocarbons. *Pharmacol.* **10** : 193.

Gillette, J. R., Plitchell, J.R. and Brodie, B. B. 1974. Biochemical mechanisms of the drug toxicity. *Annu. Rev. Pharmacol.* **14** : 271.

CHAPTER 17

HISTOPATHOLOGICAL AND BIOCHEMICAL CHANGES IN OCHRATOXICOSIS IN POULTRY (BROILERS AND COMMERCIALS)

DR. M. Vikram Reddy,
Associate Professor, Department of Pathology, CVSs,
Rajendranagar, Hyderabad - 500 030

INTRODUCTION

The importance of mycotoxins and their signficance in the health problems of man and livestock have been brought to light more in recent years, only after 1960 when there was an outbreak of turkey X disease. Mycotoxins are actually group of metabolites elaborated by fungi in the media in which they grow.

A series imporant of mycotoxins named collectively as ochratoxins are produced by the species of *Aspergillus* genera. Ochratoxin-A was first described as a toxic metabolite by Vandermerve *et al.,* (1965a).

Ochratoxin producing fungi are reported to contaminate a wide variety of feed and feed stuffs including black and red peppers, dry fish, rice, corn and peanuts. Reports reveal that *A. ochraceus* contamination is very frequent in India especially in southern region. Warehouse samples in Tamil Nadu and from the maize samples obtained from different poultry feed factories in Hyderabad have also revealed the presence of ochratoxin.

Review of literature

Effect on growth: Peckham *et al.* (1971) noticed acute toxicity of ochratoxin A and B in chicks. Daily doses of 100 ug ochratoxin A (OA) killed the birds on second day whereas daily doses of 100 ug ochratoxin B failed to kill. Sublethal doses of both toxins produced growth depression proportional to the dose.

Huff *et al.*(1974) reported that by feeding graded doses of ocharatoxin (0.5, 1.0, 2.0, 4.0 and 8.0 ug/g) in feed, form hatching until 3 weeks of age resulted in the decreased growth rate.

Prior and Sisodia (1978) found in WLH hens that by feeding 0.5, 1 or 4 ppm ochratoxin A, egg production and feed consumption declined while egg and body weights were depressed only at higher dosages. Huff and Doerr (1980) observed synergism of ocharatoxin A and aflatoxin in broiler chicken. Body weight of co-intoxicated birds were significanlty lower as against control of 2 weeks of age.

The effect of ochratoxin A on growth response was proportional to the level of exposure and was also found to be prolonged in male broilers than in females (Prior *et al.*,1980), while Reichman *et al.* (1982) reported that feeding 1 mg. kg OA for 3 weeks did not effect the conversion ratio and body weights.

Campbell *et al.*(1987) and Huff *et al.*(1983) found that by feeding aflatoxin and OA significantly decreased in body weights.

The other workers like Tohala (1983) and Kubena *et al.*(1983) Manning and Wyatt (1984) also found that by feeding OA reduces the body weight of gains significantly in laying hens as well as in broiler chicken.

Haematological changes

Rupic *et al.* (1978) reported that OA in feed at 3 ppm caused a decrease in haematocrit value, but erythrooiesis was unaffected while leucopenia in chicks was noticed.

Ochratoxin A induced iron deficiency anemia and that by iteself dose not cause haemorrhagic anemia in chicks but it elicits anaemia by causing nutritional deficiency (Huff *et la.,* 1979).

Chang *et al.* (1979) reported that OA induced marked leukopenia and monocytopenia and thus affects the immune system. It also affects phagocytic capacity of heterophils (Chang and Hamilton 1980) and thymus was regressed more rapidly (Chang *et al.*,1981). Hamilton *et al.* (1982) reported air saculitis in several field outbreaks of ochratoxicosis in broiler fowls which was due to the immuno suppressive effects of the toxin.

Goss and histopathological lesions: Vandermeve *et al.* (1965a) observed retardation of sexual maturity and low egg production in the week-old WLH chicken fed with OA with at higher concentration in addition to the above changes hepatic and renal disorders, suppression of haemopoiesis and the depletion of lymphoid elements in the spleen and bursa of fabricius were more marked in chicks. The other lesions were catarrhal enteritis with heterophilic infiltration, localised necrosis in renal tubules and urate deposition in the ureters.

Threon *et al.* (1965) noticed extensive fatty vacuolation, changes in the matrix of the mitochondria and disorganization of the endoplasmic reticulum in hepatocyts in ducklings. Doupnik and Peckham (1970) and Peckham *et al.* (1971) observed postmortem changes in WLH cockerels in ochratoxicosis. Predominantly there was visceral gout, and few petechial haemorrhages in the preventriculus and enteritis. Histopathological changes were nephrosis, hepatic degeneration and suppression of haematopoiesis.

Huff *et al.*(1974) reported enlarged kidneys and reduced growth rates were constant findings in broiler chicken. The other pathological changes were petechiae in proventriculus, gizzard erosions, pale kidney, liver and pancreas, impaired renal function and increased uric acid production. Huff *et al.*(1975) concluded that OA in young broiler chicken was mainly a nephrotoxin.

Warren and Hamilton (1981) detected glycogen storage disease type X caused by OA in broiler chickens. Affected birds showed histopathologically glycogen accumulation in muscle tissues.

Hamilton *et al.*(1982) reported air succulitis in several field outbreaks of ochratoxicosis in broiler fowls and this related to the immunosuppressive effects of the toxin.

Dwivedi and Burns (1984) recorded renal, liver and proventricular enlargement while thymus and bursa of fabricius were regressed. There was increased accumulation of cytoplasmic glygogen in hepatocytes, abnormal mitochondrial ring formation in kidneys in OA in young broiler chicks. The severity of the changes was found to be dose-related and also suggest that the mitochondria in PCT in kidney were more sensitive to OA toxicity.

Bodnarchak and Kasprak (1984) reported the presence of haemorrhages in various tissues and catarrhal gastritis and enteritis in ducks.

Manning and Wyatt (1984) observed pale friable livers, enlarged pale kidneys and gall bladders in broiler chicks in ochratoxicosis.

Brown *et al.* (1984) found that feeding of OA from 1 to 21 days of age was associated with proximla tubular, intro-nuclear bound inclusion, elongated tortuous and ring-shaped mitochondria, enlarged mitochondrial micical granules with hyaline centres and an increase in size and membrane of peroxisomes of secondary lyposomes

Subramaniam *et al.* (1986) found on PM examination of chicks in ochratoxicosis, necrosis of the liver with mild fatty changes, periportal fibrosis and fatty vacuolation. Kidneys showed nephrosis, fatty changes in distal tubules and fragmentation of glomerular capillaries. Necrosis of intestinal will was also observed

Biochemical changes: Pitout and Nell (1969) studied the inhibitory effect of OA on caroxy peptidase and found that there was an increase in the glycogen content of rate liver and a disturbance of glycogen metabolism. Thus the toxin influences both carbohydrate and protein metabolism.

Prior and Sisodia (1978) observed in OA in WLH hens that total serum proteins were decreased after feeding 1 to 4 ppm for 6 weeks.

Huff *et al.* (1979) found decreased glycogen mobilization during ochratoxicosis in broiler chickens, liver glycogen levels were raised significantly at 4 and 8 ug/g of feed.

Page *et al.* (1980) reported that ochratoxicosis leads to increased serum uric and acid levels.

Kubena *et al.*(1983) found that serum uric acid levels were significantly increased in OA and OA tannic acid combination group indicated imparied renal excretory function. Manning and Wyatt (1984) reported a significant increase in uric acid concentration in chicks fed with all forms of OA.

Subramaniam and Govindaswamy (1985) found that OA increased blood glucose levels and reduced the activities of hexokinase and aldolase in one-day chicken. These effects might be due to combination of reduced glucose oxidation and glycogen synthesis and enhanced glycoeogenesis during ochratoxicosis.

Haematological, blood glucose and uric acid and histopathological investigations were carried out in chicks fed with ochratoxin at 0.75 mg/kg body weight and 1.5 mg/kg body weight over a period of 8 weeks at the department of pathology.

The haematological investigations showed that there is significant (P/0.01) decrease in PCV, HB, total RBC count, total leucocytic count and differential counts in toxin (0.75 mg/kg body weight)-fed birds are against controls, there was further significant drop in all these values with a higher dosage of toxin.

The blood glucose values and uric acid values increased

significantly (P/0.01) in toxin fed groups when compared with control, however, there was no significant difference in these values between the two levels of toxin feeding.

There was no gross lesions in the internal organ, except congestion of the intestine at lower dosage, while at a higher dosage, the kidneys were slightly enlarged and congested and intestines and slightly haemorrhagic. The other organs did not show any change.

Histopathological changes in liver include slight to moderate congestion of central veins, simusoids and varied degrees of hepatic cell degeneration and vocuolation. Nodular lymphoid agregates were noticed in birds fed with 0.75 mg/kg body weight while these changes were still advanced in birds fed with higher levels at toxin.

In kidney-thickened basement membrance of glomeruli and fragmentation of the glomerular capillaries due to degeneration of the glomerular endothelium were noticed. Degenerative changes in the epithelium lining the proximal convoulted tubules and occasionally few hyaline casts were noticed at a lower level of toxin feeding, while these changes were much advanced at a higher level of toxin feeding.

REFERENCES

Bodnarchuk, A. I. and Kasprak, J. M. 1984. Ochra toxicosis in ducks. Path. Abstr. 19(5) : 1092 (Abstr.)

Brown, T. P., Manning, P. O., Fletcher, O. J., Wyatt, R. D. 1986. The individual and combined effects of citrinin and ochratoxin A on renal structure on layer chicks. Avian Dis. 30 : 191-198.

Campbell, M. L. (Jr.), May, J. D., Huff, W. E. and Doerr, J.A. 1983. Evaluation of immunity of young broiler chickens during simultaneous aflatoxicosis and ochratoxicosis. Poult. Sci., 62 : 2138-2144.

Chang, C. F., Doerr, J. A. and Hamilton, P. B. 1981. Comparative study of T.S. toxin ochratoxin and aflatoxin in broiler chicken. Poult Sci. 60 : 114-119.

Chang, C. F. and Hamilton, P. B. 1980. Impairment of phagocytosis by heterophils from chicken during ochratoxicosis. Applied and Environmental Microbiology, 39 : 572-575.

Chang, C. F., Huff, W. E. and Hamilton, P. B. 1979. A leucocytopenia induced in chicken by dietary ochratoxin. Poult Sci. 58 : 555-58.

Doupnik. B. and Peckham, J. O. 1970. Mycotoxicity of *Aspergillus Ochreceus* to chicks, Apply Microbiol. 19 : 594-97.

Dwivedi, P., Burns, R. B. 1984. Pathology of ochratoxicosis in young broiler chicks, Res. Vety. Sci. 36 : 92-103.

Hamilton, P. B. Huff , W. E. Havis, Jr. and Wyatt. R. D. 1982. Pathology of ochratoxin in broiler fowls, Poult Sci. 16 : 1832-1841.

Huff. W. E. and Chang, C. E., Warren, M. E. and Hamilton, P. B. 1979. Ochratoxin A induced from liron deficiency anaemia. Applied andenviron, Microbiol., 37 : 601-604.

Huff, W. E. and Doerr, J. A. 1980. Synergisu of Ochratoxin A aflatoxin in broiler chickens. Poult Sci., 59 : 1623.

Huff. W. E., Doerr, J. A., Wabeck, C. J. Chaloupka. G. W., May, J. D. and Merkeley, J. W. 1983. Individual and combined effects of aflatoxin and ochratoxin A on bruising in broiler chickens. Poult Sci., 62 : 1764-1771.

Huff, W. E., Wyatt, R. D., Tucker, T. L. and Hamilton, P. B. 1974. Ochratoxicosis in the broiler chicken. Poult Sci. 53 : 1585-1591.

Huff, W. E., Wyatt, R. D. and Hamilton, P. B. 1975. Nophatoxicity of dietary ochratoxin A in broiler chicken. Appl. Microbiol. 30 : 48-51.

Kubene, L.F., Phillips, T.D., Cregar, C.E., Witzel, D.A. and Heidelbaough, N.D. 1983. Toxicity of the Ochratoxin A and tannic acid in growing chicks. Poult Sci. 62 : 1786-1792.

Manning, R. O. and Wyatt, R. D.,1984. Toxicity of *Aspergillus ochraceus* contaminated wheat different chemical form of ochratoxin A in broiler chickens. Poult Sci. 68 : 458-465.

Page, R. K., Steward, G., Wyatt, R. D., Bush, P., Fletcher, O. J. and Brown, J. 1980. Influence of own levels of ochratoxin A on egg production, egg shall stains and serum uric acid levels in leghorn type hens. Avian Dis. 24 : 777-780.

Peckhan, J. C., Doupnic, B. and Jones, O. H. 1971. Acute toxicity of ochratoxin A and B in chicks, Apply. Microbiol. 21 : 492-494.

Pitout, M. J. and Nell, W. 1969. Inhibotory effect of ochratoxin A on bovine carboxy perptidase a in vitro, Bichem, Pharmac., 18 : 1837-1848.

Prior, G. O., Neil, J. B. and Sisodia, C. S. 1980. Effect of ochratoxin A on growth response and residues in broilers. Poult. Sci. 59 : 1254-1257.

Prior, M. G. and Sisodia, C. S. 1978. Ochratoxicosis in white leghorn hens. Poult Sci. 57 : 619-623.

Reichmann, K. G.Blancy, B. J., Conner, J. K. and Runge, B.M. 1982. The significance of aflatoxin and ochratoxin in the diet of Australian chickens, Aust, Vet. J. 58 : 211-212.

Rupic, V., Liker, B., Muzic, S., Bodganic, C., Balžer, J. 1978. Influence of ochratoxin A in feed on the blood picture of chicks, Vet. Bull., 48 : 589.

Subramaniam, S. Kanthaswamy, S., William, S. and Govindaswamy, S. 1986. Studies on the toxic nature of ochratoxin A in chicks, Indian J. Poult Sci., 21 : 354-356.

Subramaniam, S. and Govindaswamy, S. 1985. Aspergillus ochraceus toxicity and carbohydrate metabolism in chicks. Current Sci. 54 : 860-862.

Threon, J. K., Vandermerve, K. J., Liehenberg, H. J. B., Jowhert and W. Neil., 1965. Acutr liver injury in ducklings and rates as a result of ochratoxin poisoning. J. Pathol. Bacterial. 91 : 521-529.

Tohala, S. H. 1983. A study of ochratoxin toxicity of laying hens. Dissertation Abstracts international B. 44 : 655.

Vandermerve, K. J., Steyn, P.S., Fourie, S. 1965a. Mycotoxins part II. The constitution of ochratoxins, A, B and C metabolites of aspergillus ochraceus cited by Chowdhary, H., Carlson, C.W., Semenuk, G. 1971. A study of ochratoxin toxicity of hens. Poult Sci., 6 : 1855-1859.

Warren, M. F. and Hamilton, P. B. 1980. Inhibition of the glycogen phospharylase system during ochratoxicosis in chickens. Appl. and Environment Microbiol 40 : 522-525.

CHAPTER 18

ASPERGILOSIS INFECTION AND AFLATOXICOSIS IN POULTRY FEED AND ITS CORRELATION WITH VARIOUS DISEASE PROBLEMS IN POULTRY FARMS

Dr. D. Mahendranath

Technical Advisor Laboratories VHL Diseases Diagnostic Lab

Venkateshwara Hatcheries Limited, King Kothi, Hyderabad - 29

Aspergillosis

Aspergillosis or brooder penumonia is a disease mainly of respiratory system caused by inhalation of spores of Aspergillus species e.g., *Aspergillus fumigatus.*

The egg surface gets contaminated some times by the droppings, The spores germinate, hyphae travel through egg shell pores when there is moisture and colonized inside the eggs specially on the airspace membrance. Undetectable air cracks are more suitable for such fungus colonization. When these fungus contaminated eggs break in the incubators, unfortunately, the spores may be inhaled by the newly-hatchout chicks. Day-old chicks most commonly contact the disease from uncleaned, unfumigated chick guards, brooders, feeders, and curtains, and also during the transportation from the chick van. Both young and old birds contact disease by inhalation of spores developed in the feed getting wet and leftovers unnoticed for long time.

Signs

The affected birds show gasping and accelerated breathing through open beak but there are seldom rales, which occur in other respiratory diseases.

Lesions

The common lesion is formation of nodules which may be a few or many completely occupying the lungs. More common in older birds are plague-like lesions of the air sacs. Some lesions simulate the fungus colony seen on the culture plate are observed on the air sacs.

The diagnosis depends on the microscopic demonstration of fungus, and confirmation by cultural examination. The nodule may be cut and pressed into sabouraund's medium. After 48 hours typical Aspergillus colonies appear. Characteristic reproductive mycelium can be demonstrated under the microscope from these colonies to confirm the disease.

Fumigatin of shed, equipement used for brooding and curtains can control Aspergillosis (0.6 g of pot, permanganate + 1.2 ml formaldehyde/cft.)

Aflatoxicosis

Production problems in poultry, associated with feed contamination results in great economic losses yearly. Of the overall feed contamination problem, contamination due to mycotoxins represent a high percentage.

Mycotoxins which cause heavy economic losses are Aflatoxins, Trichotecenes, Ochratoxins, Citrinins, Trichotecines are produced by Fusarium sp. The ability to produce citrinins and ochratoxins are widely among Aspergillus and Pencillium species.

The moulds responsible for the production of aflatoxin are primarily *Aspergillus flavus* and *Aspergillus parasiticus.* During the growth of mould of storage grains as well as on crops, seventeen metabolic byproducts are produced, which are toxic, and are designated as Aflatoxins. But the term 'Aflatoxin' is usually referred to four compounds designated B_1, B_2, G_1 and G_2. of these B_1 is usually found in highest concentration and is the most toxic followed by G_1, B_2 and G_2.

Aflatoxin-producing moulds are primarily storage fungi but can also grow on crops in the field prior to the harvest. In general, these moulds enter the grains the harvest but in the case of groundnut the moulds infect during harvest. As the moulds grow, several metabolic byproducts are produced within the grains, without much evidence from the surface. The factors responsbile for mouldiness are:

(i) A moisture content below 12% in maize. 11% in soyabean and 10% in groundnut prevents invasion of storage fungi regardless of how long the grain is stored. If the environmental humidity is high, then moisture content of grain must be lessened. In India, groundnut, especially the winter crop, suffers from high humidity becomes loose and plants can be easily pulled out.

When harvested, nuts are stored without complete drying, the condition for mould growth becomes ideal.

(ii) A temperature range of 40° to 25°C is ideal for fungal growth, which is available in tropical, semitropical areas.

(iii) When the grains are cracked or broken during harvest by insects, they become mouldy faster than whole kernels as the coat is protective.

(iv) Drought condition is more favourable in mouldiness. The degree of susceptibility of aflatoxin is influenced by the following general factors such as:

(a) Age - young are more susceptible

(b) Sex Cockrels are more prone

(c) Health status of the bird- susceptibility increase when the birds are weak/debilitated under stress.

(d) Breeders are more susceptible than commercial layers.

There is no safe level of aflatoxin. Risks directly depend on the levels of the aflatoxins and also presence of other mycotoxins in the feed. For all practical purposes a level upto 0.03 ppm in the feed of layers may be taken as 'Safe'. Mycotoxins (Aflatoxins) in high and persistent level in poultry feed have proved to lead to immuno-suppressions and may show back down of immunity, hence it is essential to monitor feed for aflatoxins.

Symptoms and lesions of aflatoxin that could be seen in the field are:

(a) Drop in feed consumption

(b) Decreased growth rate and delayed sexual maturity

(c) Decreased egg production/weight gain

(d) Pale birds

(e) Ascitis

(f) Liver damage, which may be seen as fatty liver, fragile liver, hard liver

(g) More leg problems due to impaired calcium and phosphorus metabolism

(h) Lack of response to the treatment given for diseases like cocccidiosis, worms, disease of bacterial origin

(i) Bleeding all over the muscles

(j) Increased incidence of viral disease for which vaccination was conducted.

Symptoms and lesions which are expected to be present but go unnoticed are:

(1) Loose droppings

(2) Altered protein and energy metabolism

(3) Choking sounds in the flock

(4) White dusty comb as if sprayed with flour and shrinkage of comb

(5) Moulting in layers

(6) Enlarged gall bladder

(7) Enteritis

(8) Catarrhal exudate in deoudenum

The effect of aflatoxin on weight gain/egg production is reversible but very slow.

To minimise chances of mould contamination, the farmer should provide good conditions during harvest, transportation and storage of feed stuff. To mention some of the preventive measures:

(1) Exposure of ingredients/feed to sunlight for 1 to 2 days to reduce moisture content.

(2) One can easily find out damaged grains with naked eye as blackish/green spots of fungus seen on the grains. If one spots 100 contaminated grains in a kilo gram maize, reject the whole lot

(3) Regularly examine prepared and feed ingredients for aflatoxin content to understand the quality of material one has..

(4) Clean feeders with scrapers every week regularly and before feeding check the condition of feeders and feed in feeders.

(5) Do not store the feed longer than a week

(6) Minimise ammonia level in the poultry shed and decrease the ambient temperature

(7) The store house of feed should be 'pukka' (concrete) building free of dampness

(8) There should be cross-ventilation for feed store house.

The adverse effect of Aflatoxin is counteracted

(a) Withdrawal of feed when the toxin is high or dilute the feed ingredients so that toxin is far below safe level.

(b) Detoxify the feed even the toxin is at low level if the feed has to be used.

(c) Strengthen the liver with herbal preparation

(d) Use preparations to increase the feed consumption

(e) Increase the protein, methionine and lysine, choline chloride, vitamins (fat soluble and water soluble) selenium and biotin.

CHART SHOWING THE DATA OF AFLATOXIN ANALYSIS CONDUCTED AT VENKATESWARA HATCHERIES CITY LAB FROM 21.6.1988 TO 12.3.1990

Sample	No. of samples analaysed	Aflatoxin +Ve	Alatoxin -Ve	Range of presence of toxin in +ve samples
Compounded feed	211	102	109	0.02 ppm to 0.4 ppm
G.N. cakes	169	94	75	0.1 ppm to 0.8 ppm
Fish	32	10	22	0.1 ppm to 0.2 ppm
Maize	41	11	30	0.1 ppm to 0.4 ppm
Liver meal	9	9	0	0.1 ppm to 0.8 ppm
Meat meal	2	2	0	0.4 ppm in both
Bajra	7	3	4	0.1 ppm to 0.2 ppm
Soyabean meal	5	4	1	0.1 ppm to 0.2 ppm
Till cake	2	0	2	Below 0.05 ppm
Sunflower cake	2	2	0	0.1 ppm to 0.2 ppm
Total	480	237	243	

CHAPTER 19

AFLATOXICOSIS AND IMMUNORESPONSE IN POULTRY

Dr. S.M. Mohiuddin

Associate Professor & Head, Department of Pathology Veterinary College, Rajendranagar, Hyderabad.

INTRODUCTION

The term immunity denotes a state of relative resistance of infection. The immune system is controlled by special lymphoid organs termed Bursa of Fabricius and Thymus, the former is the source of B-cells and the latter is for T-cells

Synthesis, assembly and reaction of immunoglobulins in addition to cell mediated immuno-response (CMI) forms fascinating immune mechanism. In plasma cells (provided with radioactive amino acids). Immunoglobulins in general like other secreted proteins, are synthesized on polyribosomes attached to rough endoplasmic reticulum. The newly synthesized immunoglobulin molecules are secreted from the cells after 20-30 min, lag during which they pass through cisternae of endoplasmic reticulum, traverse the Golgi apparatus and then move towards the cell surface membrane and release Ig. molecules. During this migration the completed chains are assembled into molecules the interchain S.S. bonds are formed and sugars are added by hexotransferases to form the oligosaccharide groups of Ig. molecule.

Immunosuppression occurs due to interference with antibody formation and non-specific immunosuppression. The non-specific immunosuppressive agents, suppress cell divison or destroy lymphocytes (X-rays, radio mimetic alkalating agents).

Several etiological agents can impair the immune mechanism causing immunosuppression, of which aflatoxin are much concerned since their contamination in food grains is now well recognized as a public health hazard (Goldblatt 1971). Aflatoxin are the metabolic products of the fungus *Aspergillus flavus* and parasiticus, and has been encountered in several agricultural commodities and more so in oilseeds (Goldblatt, 1969) and animal products like meat, milk and eggs (Ramsay Tainsh, 1975).

Aflatoxins assume a greater importance than other toxins, since, apart from their hepatotoxic and immunosuppressive effects, they are animiototic (Green, 1968), teratogenic, mutagenic and carcinogenic (Ligator, 1979) in action.

Aflatoxins cause immunosuppression in the followng ways:

1. Inhibition of RNA polymerase in vivo
2. Enhanced degradation of antibodies
3. Inhibition of processing in the antigen
4. Inhibition of function of specific immunological tissue

Aflatoxins are potent immunosuppresants in the young chicken and the extent of suppression of HA response is dose-dependent and the duration of exposure. Several alternative explanations put forward are as follows:

(a) Aflatoxin has been demonstrated to inhibit RNA polymerase in vivo, and subsequently to limit protein synthesis. Immunosuppression by aflatoxin then would result in the inhibition of synthesis of specific immunoglobulins.

(b) Increased degradation of antibodies would account for immuno suppression. Aflatoxin causes rapid and dramatic increase in the specific activity of lysosomal enzymes in skeletal muscles and liver of chicken and dose-related decrease in tissue strength and integrity (Gung *et al.*1971). Since lysosomes and their hydrolytic enzymes are involved in the extra cellular and intracellular digestion of macromolecules, aflatoxin would be immunosuppressive by virtue of its ability to stimulate lysosomal degradation of immunoglobulins.

(c) Inhibition of process of antigen (immunosuppression) : The inhibiton of reticuloendothelial system by aflatoxin is a dose-dependant action. The phagocytic cells are possibly involved in the processing of the antigen.

(d) Inhibition of the specific immunological tissues is also responsible. The different kind of immunological system in chicken is dependent on the bursa fabricius for initiating cell related antibodies. It should be noted that the regression of bursa and suppression of HA response occurs with concentration of aflatoxin that does not inhibit growth. Since the potential lymphoid tissue to produce antibodies is dependent on bursa and thymus and the regression of these two organis by aflatoxin would be expected to result in impaired immunological performance.

Review of literature

Effect of aflatoxin on humoral immunity

Brown and Abram (1965) consistently isolated salmonelia from ducklings and chickens with typical aflatoxicosis. Aflatoxins are responsible for hypoproteinemia which included low levels of globulins. Thus aflatoxicosis made birds more susceptible to salmonella infection.

In rates aflatoxin appears to exert their primary effects on ribonucleic acid (RNA) polymerase as a result of binding to desoxyribonucleic acid (DNA) (Clifford and Rees, 1967 : Pong and Wagen, 1969).

Galikeev *et al.,*(1986) reported a marked depression in antibody formation in mice, when aflatoxin was given before or during the vaccination period and a moderate depression when aflatoxin was given after vaccination.

Lafarge and Frayssinet (1970) observed that aflatoxin have been shown to inhibit RNA polymerase in vivo and subsequently limit protein synthesis, resulting in immunosuppression, due to inhibition of the synthesis of specific immunoglobulins.

Pier and Heddleston (1970) studied the effect of aflatoxin on immunity in turkeys in terms of impairment of actively acquired resistance to bacterial challenge. They observed that aflatoxin B_1 0.25-0.5 ppm consumed during or after the period of immunization of manifestation of acquired resistance in 20-67% of turkey poults and chicken. Aflatoxin consumed immediately before the immunizing period did not impair the development of solid imune response. When a aflatoxin-free ration was fed for 3 weeks, after toxin consumption, weight loss and histopathological changes induced, returned to normal but the defect in immunity remained as it was when the recepients had been immunized during the period of aflatoxin consumption.

Thaxton and Hamilton (1971) reported the dose-related decrease in the ability of chicken to form haemagglutins during the aflatoxicosis, and the possible explanation for immunosuppression was explained as an impairment of the RES, which was responsible for the removal and processing of sheep red blood cells used as antigen.

Aflatoxins are reported to reduce the resistance against infection in *Candida, albican, Eimeia tenella* and Marek's diseases (Edds *et al.*,1973).

Thaxton *et al.* (1974) have shown that feeding graded levels of aflatoxin 0.625, 1.25, 5.0 and 10.0 ug/g feed from hatching signifcantly (P/0.05) depressed haemaglutination. Response at 3, 6, 9 days, after sheep red blood cells (SRBC) injection, and the degree of immunosuppression is directly related to the concentration of the dietary aflatoxin.

Tung *et al.*(1975) reported a decrease in serum IgG of chicken-fed aflatoxin 2.5 ug/g of diet, could be due to the aflatoxin or its metabolites binding randomly to template to DNA and inhibits the larger transcribing units, such as those of serum albumin and lipid before the smaller transcribing units are inhibited.

Giambone *et al.* (1978) have studied the effect of aflatoxin on humoral and CMI system of chickens. A significant decrease in serum immunoglobulins (IgG and IgA) but not in TgM, in chicks fed aflatoxins, 2.5 ug/g feed from hatching to 4 weeks of age. The deficiency of IgG immunoglobulins, an extremely important, in nuetralising infective agent, could result in increased suscepitibility to common poultry pathogens. Since, IgA is responsible for local immunity, reduction in synthesis of IgA could increase the susceptibility of chicken to local infections. The abence of IgM conc, to a marked level in chickens can be explained by the ontogency of IgM in chickens. IgM are produced during later stages of embryonic life. Therefore, aflatoxin fed to newly-hatched chicks will be too late to impair IgM producing cells.

Another important observation that aflatoxins had no residual effect on immunity. The damage produced by aflatoxin is temporary.

Since only minimal microscopic changes were noticed in various lymphoid tissues, the mechanism of immunity suppression is not by destroying the B and T cells, but by altering their function. The impairment of IgG and IgA production could result indirectly from an effect on T cells since, it has been shown that an inteact thymus is necessary for switchover production from IgM and IgA producing cells. Impairment of T cell function or maturation by aflatoxin could explain the deficiency in IgC and IgA production.

Mohiuddin *et al.*,(1981) reported that chickens fed with 0.2 ppm of aflatoxin over a period of 21 days had depressed antibody titres significantly (P/0.01) against Raniket disease vaccines.

Reddy *et al.* (1983) have studied the dose and time-related responses of immunological function in young adult mice fed 0, 30, and 700 ug/kg weight of aflatoxin B_1. A decrease in homoral immunity at both the primary and secondary antibody response was noticed.

Panaugala *et al.*(1986) studied the effect of aflatoxin in pigs and reported that humoral response was not affected, however, a significant reduction was noticed in complement titres and an increase in serum IgG, IgM value on feeding 560 ug/kf of feed.

Balaraman and Arora (1987) suggesed that binding of aflatoxin to immunoglobulin molecules reduced their absorption thereby the serum levels were decreased.

Purified aflatoxin even @ 0.25 ug/g when fed to birds from second day of age, lowered the protection rate against fowl pox virus (Sharma, 1988).

Effect of aflatoxin on cellular immunity

Micheal *et al.* (1973) studied the effect of graded doses of dietary aflatoxicosis (0, 0.625, 1.25, 2.5 and 5.0 ug) on the functions of reticulo endothelial system, in clearing colloidal carbon from circulation. The rate of clearance was found to have decreased significant (P/0.05) at 1.25 ug/g of diet. The data indicated clearly that reticuloendothelial systems is impaired seriously and so the primary defence barrier against foreign matter is broken and thus presumably a decreased ability to process the antigenic complets.

Chang *et al.* (1976) have reported that the chemotactic activity of heterophils to phagocytose was markedly reduced in chickens fed a diet containing 2.5 ug of aflatoxin/g feed, reflecting upon the impairment of cellyular immunity.

Giambone *et al.*(1978) reported that chickens fed 2.5 ug of aflatoxin/g diet during 2-4 weeks of age or from hatching to 84 weeks were deficient in CMI, measured at 4 weeks of age by graft versus host reaction.

Richard *et al.*(1983) studied the effect of feeding corn naturally contaminated with aflatoxin on feed efficiency and immunological changes in steers. There was a delayed cutaneous hypersensitivity when fed aflatoxin at 800 ug/ g feed.

Bodine *et al.*(1984) have reported the effects of aflatoxin B_1 and major metabolites on phytohaemagglutinins stimulated lymphoblastogenesis in bovine lymphocytes. It was observed that moderate to strong inhibition of blastogenesis resulted in inhibition of T-lymphocytes function such as killer, helper, effector or other immunological process.

Ozean (1984) studied histomeric and histomorphological studies on the effect of aflatoxin on plasma cells in chickens. Ten 4 month old chicks were given aflatoxin in their drinking water for four successive days (total dose of 0.22 mg aflatoxin B_1). On the fifth day there were vaccinated against Newcastle disease and along with them controls given vaccine only. There were killed on seer or 15 days later. In chicks pyrinophilic cell count and electron microscopy of plasma cells in the small intestine, spleen, thymus and bursa fabricius were treated in aflatoxin-fed chicken but not prevented the development of immunity.

Sinha and Arora (1984) have studied the influence of aflatoxin and disease incidence and in vivo response of lymphocytes nitrogen in kids and found a decreased immunological response.

Visalkshen *et al.* (1984) studied the effects of natphthyl acetate activity in lymphocytes in pigs and found that the total lymphocytic count were reduced while erythropoietic activity was not affected.

Giambone *et al.* (1985) studied the effects of purified aflatoxins-on broiler chickens and turkey. CMI response was measurted by delayed type of hypersensitivity reaction was significantly affected in birds receiving 400 ppg of pure aflatoxin B_1 and B_2.

Aflatoxin suppresses in vitro bovine and caprine lymphocytic response to phytomytogens (Sinha and Arora, 1985).

Mohiuddin *et al.* (1986) studied the phagocytic activity in aflatoxin fed chicken. It was reported that the phagocytic activity of heterophils and kupffer cells was markedly depressed.

Thurstan *et al.* (1986) studied the effects of aflatoxin given in single or multiple doses in cattle. In single dose animals, complement activity and bacteriostatic activities decreased but returned to normal by 168 hrs. However, in multiple dose animals only the bacteriostatic activity decreased and persisted for two weeks. Apparently aflatoxins affect both complement-dependent and independent serum bacteriostatic activity.

Reddy *et al.* (1987) studied the immune function of CD-1 mice exposed to aflatoxin B1 and observed that the synthesis of DNA was decreased in lymphocyte cultures antibody production by splenic cells in animals challenged with T dependent antigen (sheep RBC), was affected by aflatoxin B1, while no effects were noticed when challenged with T independent antigen.

CONCLUSION

From the review of available literature, it is evident that aflatoxin impair phagocytic activity of macrophages, monocytes and heterophils (Mechiel *et al.*,1973 : Chang *et al.*, 1976) depress IgG and IgA (Giambone *et al.*, 1978) impairs CMI response, leucocyte migration inhibit phytohaemagglutinin stimulaters, lymphoblastogeneses, interferon production (Pier and Heddleston, 1970 : Bodine *et al.*, 1984) and complement fixation (Chang *et al.*, 1976) in serum.

Aflatoxin also affect the reticulo endothelial system. Whether the immunosuppression is temporary and reversible is not well established, which needs further investigation.

The immunosuppressive effect of aflatoxin in cel mediated as well as humoral immune system is well documented in poultry. Such studies need to be carried out in other species of livestock.

REFERENCES

Brown, J.M. and Abrams, L. 1965. Biochemical studies on aflatoxicosis. Onertepoort, J. Vet. Res. **32** : 119-146.

Bodine, A.B., Fisher, S.T., Gangjee, S. 1984. Effect of aflatoxin B_1 and major metabolism and phytohaemagglutinin stimulated lymphoblastogensis of bovine lymphocytes. J. Dairy Sci. **67** : 110-114.

Balaraman, N. and Arora, S.P. 1987. Effect of aflatoxin on imunoglobulin status in blood serum of neonatal calves. Indian J. Anim. Sci. **57** (1) : 62-63.

Cliford, J.I. and Rees, K.R. 1967. The action of aflatoxin B1 on the rat liver. Biochem. J. **102** : 65-75.

Chang, G.F., Hamilton, P.B. and Weeks. B.A. 1976.. Chemotaxis and phagocytosis during aflatoxicosis. Anna. Med. Anim, Sci. Microbiol. 181.

Edds, G.T., Nair, K.P.C. and Sinapsen, C.F. Amer, J. Vet. res. **34** : 819.

Galikeev, K.L., Raipovor and Manyaasheva, R.A. 1968. Effect of aflatoxin on dynamics of antibody formation. Abst. Vet. Bull.

Greens, S. 1968. Antineoplastic activity of aflatoxin B1. Nature **220** : 931-932.

Goldblatt, L. A. 1969. Aflatoxin, Scientific, background, control and implementations, P.I. Academic Press, N.Y.

Giambone, J. J., Ewert, D.L., Wyatt, R.D. and Edisow, O.S. 1978. Effect of aflatoxin on humoral cell mediated immune system of the chicken. Amer. J. Vet. Res. **39** : 305-308.

Giambone, J. J., Diener, U.L., Panaugala, V. S. and Horr, F. 1985. Effects of aflatoxin the on young broiler chiken. Poult Sci. **64** : 1678-1680.

Legator, W. B. 1961. Mutagenic effects of aflatoxin. J. Amer. Vet. Assoc., 155-2020.

Lafarge, G. and Frayssinet. G. 1970. The reversibility of inhibition of RNA and DNA synthesis induced by aflatoxin in rat liver A tentative explanation for carcinogenic metabolism. Int. J. Cancer, **6** : 74-83.

Michaelco, Y. P., Thaxton, J.P. and Hamilton, P. B. 1973. Impairment of reticulo endothelial system of chicken during aflatoxicosis, Poult Sci., **52** : 1206-1207.

Mohiuddin, S. M., Mahendranath, D., Yadagiri, B. and Ahmed, S.R. 1968. Studies on the effect on aflatoxin on antibody synthesis against Raniket disease vaccine in chicks, Indian J. Anim, Sci. **510** : 72-82.

Mohiuddin, S. M., Vikram Reddy, M. Madhava Reddy, M. and Ramakrishna, K. 1986. Studies on phagocytic activity and haematological changes in aflatoxicosis in poultry. Indian Vet. J. **63 :** 442-445.

Ozean, A. 1984. Histomeric and Histomorphological studies on the effect of aflatoxin on plasma cells in chicks. Abst. Vet. Bull No. 3114.

Pong, R. S. and Wogan, G. M. 1969. Time, course of alaterations of rate liver polysome profiles induced by aflatoxin B1. Biochem. Pharmacol. **18** : 2357-2361.

Pier, A. and Heddleston, K.L. 1970. The effect of aflatoxin on immunity on turkeys to bacterial changes. Avian Dis. **14** : 797-809.

Panaugala, V. S., Giambone, J. J., Dier, V. L., Davis, N. D., Hoerr, E. J., Miller, A., Scaucty and Wilt, G. R. 1986. Amer. J. Vet. Res. **47 (9)** : 2062-2067.

Ramsay Tainsh, A. 1975. Preliminary and secondary mycotoxicosis. Indian J. Envir. Studies **8** : 161-177.

Richard, J.L., Pier, A.C., Stubblefield, R.D., Shotwell, O.L., Lyan, R.L. and Cullip, A.C. 1983. Effect of feeding corn naturally contaminated with aflatoxin on feed efficiency, physiology and immunologic and pathologic changes and tissue residues and stern. Amer, J. Vet. **44** (9) : 1294-1299. Review Med. Vet. Myed. 18 (3) 1983.

Reddy, R. V., Sharma, R.P. , Taylor, M. J. 1983. Dose and time related response of immunologic functions to aflatoxin in micr. Develop. Toxicol. environ. Sci. **11** : 431-434. Review Med. Vet. Mycol. 20 (3), 1985.

Reddy, R. V., Taylor, M. J. and Sharma, R. P. 1987. Studies on immune function of col. mice exposed to aflatoxin B1. J. Toxicol. **43** (2) : 123-132.

Sinha, R. P. and Arora, S. P. 1984. Influence of feeding aflatoxin on disease incidence and on in vivo response of lymphocytes to nitrogen in kids. Indian J. Dairy Sci. **37** (4) : 412-414.

Sinha, R. R. P. and Arora, S.P. 1985. Indian J. Anim. Nut. 1019.

Sharma D. K. 1988. Immunosuppressive effect of aflatoxin in fowlpox virus vaccine. Poultry Nov. **30** (Vol. V(1) : 181.

Thaxton, J. P. and Hamilton, P. B. 1971. Immunosuppression in broilers by aflatoxin. Poultry Sci. **50** : 1636.

Thaxton, J. P., Tung, H. T. and Hamilton, P. B. 1974. Immunosuppression in chicks by aflatoxicosis. Poult Sci. **53** : 721-725.

Tung, H. T., Wyatt, R. D., Thaxton, P. and Hamilton, P.B. 1975. Concentration of serum proteins during aflatoxicosis. Toxicol. and Appl. Pharmacol. **34** : 320-326.

Thurston, J. R., Cook. W., Driftmier, E., Richard, J. J. and Sack, J. M. 1986. Decrease complement and bacteriostatic activity in the sera of cattle given single or multiple doses of aflatoxin. Amer J. Vet. Sci. **47** (4): 846-849.

CHAPTER

20

PATHOGENI MOULD IN POULTRY DISEASES

Dr. B.K. Panda,
Principal Scientist, Project Directorate on Poultry, Hyderabad

Fungi are the parasites with variable shape and size starting from single-celled yeast to a giant multicellular mushrooms.The usefulness of many species within the family is well known. Many diseases are known to be associated with certain moulds. Out of 50000 species (Emmons *et al.*, 1977) of fungi , only 100 species are said to be pathogenin to man, animals and birds.

Like that of the *E.coli,* most of the moulds remained as common flora in different systems of birds and lower animals. When there is upset of balance due to one or the other factors, these moulds proliferate and clinically disease is produced. The predisposing factors for their proliferation includes

1) Continue therapy with brcad spectrum antibiotics and corti-consterioids.
(2) Deficiency of vitamins like Vit.A and B
(3) High energy diet favour the growth of many moulds
(4) The toxic metabolites and enzymes produced by certain fungi damages the local tissue and helped in establishing the secondary infections.
(5) Unhygenic surrounding and mouldy feed is the main source in spreading the diseases.

The purpose of this toxic is to highlight the pathogenesis and control of important mould which produces diseases in various organs of poultry birds.

Avian condidiasis and aspergillosis are the main mycotic diseases affecting turkeys, chicken, ducks, guinea fowls, quails, partridges and other animals including man. In addition to the above the other mycotic diseases like mucormycosis, phycomycosis, rhinosporidiosis coccidiodomycosis, cryptococcosis etc. are rarely the diseases that affect the birds.

Candidiasis

Candida albican is the common fungi affecting the digestive tract the disease is known as "Thrush", "Candidiasis", Moneliasis", "Oidiomycosis", "Mycotic diarrhoea" and "Sourcrop". Young birds are most susceptible than adults. The systemic candidiasis affecting G.I. tract of poultry in India reported by Pathak and Singh (1959), Choudhury and Singh (1984) are Patnaik *et al.*(1987) in their study of mycotic diseases in poultry. It is recorded that crop mycosis is mainly associated with *C. albicans, C. krusel, C parakrusei, C. tropicallis, C. steloloides, C.ruquosa and C paraspilosis.* Out of 8 species of candida, *Calbicans* is the common pathogen for poultry birds throughout the world.

Clinical signs

The affected chicks revealed the clinical symptoms like listlessness, ruffled feathers poor consumption of feed and water resulting in the loss of body weight. nervous signs like spasmodic tremor, oipisthotoinus and toritcolis is also recorded in few causes (Sahu and Mishra, 1987). Aorta and blood vessels of turkeys are also affected by the endotoxins produced by *C. albicans* (Tripathi, 1965).

The gross lesins in chickens are mainly present in the mucosa of mouth, proventriculus, crop and intestine. The affected area is thickend and frequently corrugated like a turkish towel. The mouth and oesophagus may show ulcerations.

Histopatholgogy

Candidiasis affected crop revealed thickening of mucosa. The strutum corneaum shows hyperkeratosis and parakeratosis with hyperplasia and degenerative changes of the mucosal cells. The muscular coat becomes oedamatus. The serosal surface is thickened due to oedema and congested capillaries. In mucocutaneous candidiasis, the fungus is seen either in masses of branching septate hyphae, pseudohyphae, round to oval yeast cells are seen on the surface of epithelium. There is infiltration of heterophils and lymphocytes.

Veneral candidiasis of geese resulting inflammation necrossi of the penis and cloaca and reported in Isreal. It was controlled by mass vaccination with Ethanol killed C. albican culture by I/V or I/D route.

Cutaneous candidiasis affecting the foot pads and joints of the legs in Japanese quails has been reported by Shah *et al.* (1982) With granulomatus changes of the dermis. Candida albicansis is the causative agent.

Diagnosis

1. From clinical and gorss p.m. lesion
2. The suspected materials may be mounted with 10% KoH or lactophenol cotton blue for identification of candida species.
3. Isolation of candida species of sabouraud's dextrose agar. The young colony in culture medium is white to creamy in colour whereas, the old colony is feathery in appearance due to growh of mycelia
4. The biochemical properties of candida species included fermentation of glucose and maltose-producing acid and gas.
5. Biological test-when pathogenic strain of candida is injected I/V to rabbit and mice, abscesses formation in the kidney is noted.
6 The serological tests like immuno diffusion, counter immunoelectrophoresis, tube agglutination are employed for positive sera samples
7. By immunofluorescence technique- it can be used for the rapid detection and identification of both viable and nonviable fungi from clinical materials.

Treatment and control

Effective treatment for candidiasis can be achieved by in vitro drug sensitivity test (Shah *et al.*, 1986). However, the following drugs may be used in chicken:

1. Copper sulphate 1 g/2 lit. of drunking water (1: 2000 for 7-10 days)
2. Gentian violetor methylene blue @ 1:10,000 as feed additive for 15-20 days proved effective for control of candidiasis
3. Formic acid 6% 200 ml/kg of feed for 20 days is effective
4. Angigungal drugs like Nystatin 50-100 mg/kg of feed controls the growth of candida
5. Trichomycin 40,000 i.u/lit of drunking water for 7-10 days is also effective.
6. Bayer 5097 2 100 mg/kg body weight daily control candidiasis in chicken.

Control measures

1.Maintain good hygiene and sanitation in the poultry environment
2. Avoid addition of broad spectrum antibiotics in feed
3. Segregation of affected birds to avoid further spread of disease
4. Litter hygiene should be maintained.

Respiratory candidiasis

Respiratory candiddis is not uncommon in poultry. Sansonetti (1954) Sharma *et al.* (1970) and Singh and Singh (1971) reported candida infectionn from ganulomatous lesions of lungs.

Aspergillosis

It is primarily a disease of the respiratory system affecting most of the avian species. The disease also known as "Brooder pneumonia", "Pneumomycosis", "Mycotic pneumonia" "bronchomycosis" and "Pseudotuberculosis".

The disease is caused by *A. fumigatus, A.niger, and A. nudulans* which are morphologically characterized by branching septate hyphae 2-3 micron in diameter wtih condiophores. The spores by widely distrubuted in nature thus chicks are affected by inhalation of the aspergillus spores. The fungus also grows very well in feed, litter and other organic matters. High humidity, faulty broodind and poor nutrition predispose for and attack to chick. Contaminated egg shells may also spread the diseases during incubation.

Several reports confirmed thatapsergillus species produces toxin materials from the spores viz. haemotoxin, neurotoxic and histotoxic with variable symptoms. Avian aspergillosis has been reported since 1815 and since then, volumes of publication have been added to this disease. Asthana (1944) first recorded the incidence of aspergillosis in poultry in India. Since, then, several reports have been published by Rajan *et al.* (1965) and Babras *et al.* (1967). Sharma *et al* (1971). Rao *et al.* (1982) and Panda *et al.* (1983).

Pal and Dabiya (1984) reported dermatitis due to *A. fumigatus* infection in poultry for the first time. Daka and Rao (1985) have reported *A. nidulasn* infection in ducklings. Panda (1984) also reported aspergillosis in Japanese quails from India.

Mode of infection

The spores of aspergillus entered into the host body through inhalation. Then, the fungi grown in the lungs by penetrating the mycelia into the living cells and sets up pathologcial lesions in the invaded cells. Then the fungi is disseminated to other organis, systems through haematogenous route like kidney, liver, brain and intestine etc. These fungi also stimulate granulomatus reaction in the tissues. Outbreaks of this disease are also noted in newly-hatched chicks due to hatchery contamination and also by use of mouldy straw as litter.

Clinical signs

The clinical signs of this disease is classified into two forms viz., acute from which is mostly seen in very young chicks with high mortality. The other signs prior to death included dullness, respiratory distress, discharges from nose and yes. Keratitis and blindness is also noted in or both the eyes. Diarrhoea and prostractic condition are noted at times. Young and adult birds in actue attact developed inappetance, gasping, cyanosis of comb and wattle with foetid diarrhoea. Birds, which survive the acute attack, revealed chronic form of the disease with symtpoms of chronic respiratory diseases.

Gross postmorterm changes

Aspergillosis may be suspected in postmortem examination when greenish yellow caseous exudates are present in the lung or air sac. The infection may extend into the kidneys, liver and spleen by direct contract from the airpassages, on the GI tract mucosa with either inflammation or fibrosis. Occasionally, bunches of fungi are visible to the naked eye in the air passeges of lungs, air sac or in the abdominal cavity.

Histopathology

Tissue samples collected from lungs, brochi, liver and air sac are fixed. Adequate diagnosis of the fungal agents and characterisitic tissue changs can be detected by haematoxylin and eosin or by special stains like gram, periodica aci schiff (PAS), Gridley's fungus stain and Gomori's methanamine silver stain etc. The tissue changes in the affected area of lungs as recorded by Panda *et al.*(1983) included congestion of capillaries, with areas off necrosis. Inflammatory changes with presence of heterphils and lymphocytes in the lung parenchyma is more marked in acute cases. Chronic cases were characterized by the presence of typical granulomatus lesions. Numerous branching septate hyphae are seen in the necrosed areas.

Diagnosis

1 From the history of clinical symptoms
2. By postmortem lesions
3. By direct microscopic examination of affected tissues or by special staining procedures.
4. By cultural and animal innoculation

Treatment and control

The treatment of aspergillosis established cases is of little effective. However, in the face of an outbreak, the following treatment may be advocated to prevent further spread of the diseases.

1. Copper sulphate 1 : 2000 concentraction may be used continuoulsy for 10-15 days.
2. Potassium iodide 0.1 g/lit has been used for control measures
3. Antifungal preparations like Nystatin @ 100 g/t of feed is said to be effective during outbreak
4. Hamycin @ 20 microgram/ml of D.W. for 7 days.

Respiratory mycormylosis

This condition though rare in birds has been reported from India by Parihar (1972) from routine histopathological studies. The clinical symptoms and gross lesion are not sonprominent. However, at times, the lungs are congested with few yellowish grey foci air sacs revealed thickening, opacity with coseopurulent exudates. Microscopic lesions consist of granulomas in the lungs parenchyma. Necrotic centres are surrounded by wide zone of granulomatious inflammatory tissue comprising of epithelial cells, giant cells, lymphocytes, plasma cells and heterophils. The fungal hyphae are found in between the lesion and healty tissues.

Dermatomycosis

Fungal agents affecting the featherless parts like comb and wattle is known as Favus or white comb. The fungi *Trichophyton megnini* is commonly involved although others like *T. simiti, T. mentagorophytes* are also isolated from dermatomycosis of comb.

The lesions start with a small white rounded spot and gradually spread over the surrounding tissues giving a whitish scaly appearance as if sprinkled with flour, At times, scales may form crusts wth depresse centres.Treatment of this disease is not economical and as such birds should be disposed of for table purpose. Proper health care and hygiene is essential to control this disease.

REFERENCS

Asthana, R.P. 1944. Aspergillosis in fowl. Proc. Indian Acad. Sci. **20 : B** 43-47.

Babras, M.A., Kuduskar, S.P. and Ajinkya, S.M. 1967. Some records of outbreaks of aspergillosis in chicks in Maharashtra, Part II. Incidence in broiler chickens. Poultry Diseases Seminar. IVRI. 1967.

Choudhury, B. and Balwant Singh, B. 1984. Prevalence, Pathology and isolation studies on mycosis in domestic fowls. Indian J. Anim. Sci. **54(1)** : 84-92.

Daka, P.N. and Rao, A.T. 1985. Pathogenicity of A nidulance in day-old ducklings and chicks. Poult Advi. **29(9)** : 61-62.

Emmons, C.W., Binford, C.H., Otz., B.I.J.P. and Knwochung, K.J. 1977. Medical mycoly, 3rd Edn. Lea & Febiger, Philadelphia, USA.

Jand, S.K. and Dhillon, S.S. 1973. Respiratory diseases of poultry, fungi associated with. Indian Vet. J. **50** : 221-224.

Pal, M. and Debiya, S.M. 1984. Studies on avian dermatitis caused by A. fumigatus, Indian Vet. J. 64(3): 188-190.

Panda, B.K., Shah, R.L., Arya, S.C. and Kataria, J.M. 1983. Investigation on the outbreak of aspergillosis in White leghorn chicken. Indian J. Poult Sci. **18**: 199-202

Panda, B.K. 1984. An investigation of aspergillosis in Japanese quails. Souvenir issue and Annual Convention of the Indian Society of Veterinary Medicine, p44.

Parihar, N.S. 1972. Mycosis in poultry. Summer Institute in Avian Pathology, IVRI, Izatnagar, UP. pp 122-243.

Pathak, R.C. and Singh, C.M. 1959. Occurrence of candida species in crop of fowl. Indian J. Microbiol. **12** : 2.

Ranjan, A. , Seshadri, S.J., Chandrasekharan Nair, K.P.and Rai, B.N. 1965. Avian aspergillosis. Studies on natural cases and experimental transmission. Indina Vet. J. **42** : 390-401.

Rao, M.R.K.M., Choudhury, C. and Khan, D.I. 1982. An outbreak of acute aspergillosis in chicks, Indian Vet. J. **59(5)** : 341-342.

Patnaik, G.M., Rao, A.G., Chanda, S.K. and Dash, S.N. 1987. Candidiasis in poultry. Orissa Vet. J. **15(1)** : 63-66.

Sahoo, S. and Mishra, P.K. 1987. Candidiasis in chicken. M.V. Sc. thesis submitted to Orissa University of Agriculture and Technology Bhubaneswar 751 003.

Sah, R.L., Mall, M.P. and Mohanty, G.C. 1982.Cutaneous candiddiasis in Japanese quail *(Coturnix coturnic japonica)*. Mycopathologia **80(1)**: 33-37.

Shah, N.M., Dholkia, P.M. and Simaria, M.B., 1986. In vitro drug sensitivity trials against yeast and moulds isolated from bovine udder. Indian Vet. J. **63**: 5-8.

Sharma, V.D., Sethi, M.S. and Negi, S.K. 1971. Fungal flora of respiratory tract of fowl. Poult Sci. **50**: 1041-1044.

Singh, M.P. and Singh, C.M. 1971. Candidiasis in poultry. Indian J. Anim, Sci. **41**: 294-297.

Sharma, V.d., Sethi, M.S. and Negi, S.K. 1970. Pulmonary candidiasis in fowl. Poult Sci, **49:** 1169-71.

Tripathy, S.B. 1965. Candidiasis in Turkeys. Ph.D. thesis.

CHAPTER

21

AFLATOXICOSIS IN POULTRY

S.P. Arora,
Additional Director of Research (Anim, Sci.) H.P. Krishi Vishva Vidyalaya, Palampur - 176 062 (Himachal Pradesh)

Aflatoxins are a group of closely related toxins produced by the fungi such as *Aspergillus flavus* and *A. parasiticus.* These species may produce aflatoxin of different types such as B1, B2, G1 or G2 etc. Out of all these types, AF-B1 is most toxic has been shown to cause malignant carcinoma in troug at levels as low as 15 ppb (Eddis, 1973. Prolonged feeding of its low doses can lead to hepatic lesions and lower resistance to different diseases (Newberne, 1973 : Sinha and Arora, 1984 : Balaraman and Arora, 1985). Risk is involved to human health when its intake of aflatoxins and other mycotoxins as causative factors (Wogan, 1968). In certain countries like USA and Britain aflatoxin control programme has been initiated and maximum permissible limits have been defined (Dickens, 1977: Anon., 1981). This problem has been recognized more in countries having tropical and subtropical climates where its spread is quick (Valid *et al.*, 1981). These toxins are stable to processing and cooking and can grow on variety of feedstuffs. Chemically two classifications are known:

i) Difurocuoumardactones

ii) Difurocoumarocyclopentanones

Their strong fluorescent characteristic is due to the presence of the coumarin skeleton in their structure. Optimum temperature for its production has been reported to range from 25-30°C with moisture level of 16% in feedstuffs. Insect damage has a positive influence on its propagation. Groundnut meal, maize, wheat, linseed cake, safflower cake, sunflower cake, cotton seek cake sorghum, rice, sesame cake and many other feed stuffs have been reported to contain aflatoxins in India (Yadgiri and Tulpule, 1974 : Singh *et al.*, 1984: Reddy *et al.*, 1984 : Sinha and Arora, 1985).

Prevalence in feed stuffs

Both the species of *Aspergillus* are widespread in air and soil. Earlier work reported in this country mostly referred to aflatoxin absence or presence in feeds but lately with better techniques and instrumentation, quantative estimations are being reported (Mishra and Singh, 1978: Fulsounder and Shukla, 1978: Patel *et al.*, 1981: Singh *et al.*, 1984: Reddy *et al.*, 1984). In a single study as observed, groundnut cake contained AF-B_1 0.12 to 1.0 ppm and AF-G_1 0.08 to 0.10 ppm whereas other feed stuffs revealed AF-B_1 .04 to 1.0 ppm and AF-G_1 0.04 to 0.1 ppm (Sinha and Arora, 1985)

Their mode of toxicity is due to lactone ring in AF-B series, which is cytoxic, and have the property to react with SH groups within the cellular constituents. Opening of lactone ring or saturation of double bond in the ring leads to decrease in toxicity. Similarly dihydrofurofuranmoiety in AF-G series is toxigenic. After absorption, it causes liver damage and reduces vitamin A levels in blood plasma.

Susceptiblity

Heavery mortality was reported as early as in 1960 in ducklings, peasants and patridges as a result of feeding contaminated groundnut cake (Asplin and Carnaghan, 1961). Acutely the birds showed subcutaneous haemorrhages, increases in liver content and peripheral zone necrosis. Later Carnaghan (1965) induced hepatic carcinoma by giving 0.03 ppm AF for 14 months in Turkeys.

The cases of aflatoxicosis were reported in ducklings from India wherein the maize contained 0.28 ppm AF (Rao *et al.*,1982). chicken seem to be less suceptible as 0.6 ppm AF dose had little effect on growth or on the laying ability. Gumbmann *et al* .(1970) studied its susceptibility in 18 different strains of chicken, turkey and quail and opined that this was a genetically-controlled factor. New Hampshire chicks and turkey poults were affected at 0.8 ppm AF, but WLH cross chicks did not exhibit any susceptibility at that level, and same was true with Austrolop chicken and guinea fowl. Tung *et al.* (1972) observed that aflatoxin fed at a level of 1.25 ppm or more to chicks resulted in increased liver weight and liver lipids. In layers, there is a report of reduction in egg production of 1 pm level (Reddy *et al.*, 1984). Cockerels have been shown to decrease in weight gain at a level of 2.5 ppm AF (Shukla and Pachauri, 1985).

Effects on metabolism

Aflatoxins have been reported to affect remen microbial multiplication (Mathur *et al.*, 1976: Sinha and Arora, 1982: Balaraman and Arora, 1984) leading to different fermentation pattern and ultimately affecting the availability of essential nutrients to the host. Reduction in blood glucose and decrease of glycogen content of brain and liver are noticed commonly (Barrows *et al.*, 1978). Infusion studies with 14C-proprionate indicate that propionate is converted less into glucose in liver showing liver damage when aflatoxin is administered (Sinha and Arora, 1984). Muscles are also affected in their function as experimented using 14-C-tyrosine as an index of activity or by the use of 15N-Isotope. Muscle protein synthesis (Arora, 1988), cellular DNA and RNA synthesis in live are also adversely affected (Wragg *et al.*, 1967). Another significant inlfuence of aflatoxin toxicity is on immunity breakdown as serum immunoglobulin levels decrease with incremental increase in level of aflatoxin (Pier, 1973 : Sinha and Arora, 1984: Balaraman and Arora, 1985). In chicken, aflatoxin may affect Bursa fabricus and thymus glands and there may be poor reaction of disease resistance.

Control measures

Minimization of aflatoxin contamination could be best achieved by improving feed storage conditions. Cool, dry, aerate store space and low moisture content in the feed stuff would help a long way in reducing in the fungal growth. Contamination in usually confined to small proportion of feed stuffs, less than 1 per cent in groundnut kernels (Goldblatt, 1971). About 80 to 100 per cent of aflatoxin contamination was observed to be concentrated in 2 to 9 per cent of cottonseed (Lee *et al.*, 1977). Strong or physical separation either manually or buy ultraviolet screening can reduce the toxin level considerably without loss of the valuable feed material. Heat treatment (Mann *et al.*, 1971: Lee *et al.*, 1977), chemical treatment, especially ammoniation (Brekke *et al.*, 1978: Spothen and Clawson, 1979), microbial treatment (Ciegler *et al.*, 1966) and solvent scale treatment of contaminated feeds. Recently there is a report that aluminosilicate based compound used commerically to keep from caking has also the property of absorbing aflatoxin, which passes harmlessly through the intestinal tract (Kubena and Harvey, 1988).

Fixing limits by States

Food and Drug administration has set a maximum limit of 20

ppb in the diet of chicken, dairy cattle and human beings. But in this country experiments to elucidate such levels have not been conducted. Evidences available so far indicate that LD_{50} and tolerable limits depend upon species, age, state of health, strain and level of protein or liquid in the diet. The concern is more at present with subclinical levels, which affect production in animals and thus in turn to public health through their products. The level fixed as a uniform policy by FDA may not hold good under practical conditions when the levels encountered in feed stuffs are much higher. From time to time, relaxation is practised to cover up but without any basis.

Safe dietary levels

Very little information is available on the safe levels of AF in compound feeds for different species and to generate this information, long-term studies are necessary. Research work is important in this direction to provide norms for feed quality control. Certain reports which reveal information on this aspect have been considered for this paper as an initial step in this direction particularly in poultry. It appears as if all species may not have same toleration limits, thus in this direction certain experiments were conducted. In one experiment 108 commercial Hyline male chicks, 1 day old, form a single batch were allotted randomly to 3 groups and were fed basal diet in group 1, basal diet + 0.5 ppm AF (B_1, 0.34 ppm) in group 2 and basal diet + 1.0 ppm AF (B_1, 0.75 ppm) in group 3 for a period of 8 weeks. The growth rates were 61.27, 64.63 and 59.53 g per week calculated by regression analysis. Thus the results indicated that chicks could tolerate 1 ppm level of AF. Other parameters for comparison are as under:

	Group 1	**Group 2**	**Group 3**
No. of chicks	36	36	36
Initial weight (g)	38.14	37.54	37.40
Final wt. (g)	532.22	555.28	509.44
Weekly feed consumption/chick (g)	210.3	212.23	212.23
Weekly gain	61.27	64.63	95.53
Feed gain ratio	3.39	3.49	3.65

In another experiment, 120 broiler strain of commercial cobb chicks, one day., we randomly distributed into 3 groups. The control group 1 received basal diet whereas chicks of groups 2 and 3 were given 1 ppm and 1.5 ppm AF in addition mixed in the ration. The crude AF contained 40.4% B_1 and 41.7% G1. The total AF levels were 0.19, 1.15 and 1.71 ppm in the respective 3 diets and the final weights were 1226.39, 1211.47 and 1126.11 g respectively. The data thus indicated that broiler chicks tolerated well even 1.71ppm AF level. Other parameters for comparison are as under:

	Group 1	Group 2	Group 3
No. of chicks	40	40	40
AF dose ppm	0.19	1.15	1.71
Mortality	4	6	4
Initial weight (g)	41.75	40.85	40.97
Final weight (g) 7 w	1226.39	1121.47	1126.11
Mean growth rate (g/week)	178.51	175.35	164.48
Total feed intake (kg)	3.165	3.085	3.116
Feed efficiency	2.67	2.63	2.87

Chicken seems to be highly tolerant to AF and 1 ppm level is quite tolerable. In contrast, turkey is the species, which may not tolerate even as low 0.25 ppm AF (Pier, 1973). Looking into other species, such as 4 months aged calves and buffalo calves, toleration level is only 0.26 ppm (Arora, 1988). In neonatal kids, this limit is only 0.147 ppm. Though certain reports indicate that higher level of protein or methionine (Voige *et al.*, 1980) or fat (Shank *et al.*,1972) give protection but under normal pattern of feeding it may not be feasible. Similarly extra quantity of vitamins may also be useful to protect but again with extra cost.

In conclusion, it may be inferred that more research work is required to be carried out to fill in the gaps in the knowledge particularly with regards to toxicity pattern and toleration limits for different species and for different age groups so as to be more practical in prevention on a field scale.

REFERENCES

Anon, 1981. Fertilizers and feeding stuffs (Amendment) regulations (1981) Report Vet. Rec. 108: 154.

Asplin, F.D. and Carnaghan, R.B.A. 1961. Vet. Rec., 73 : 1215-1218.

Arora, S.P. 1988. Studies on the influence of different levels of aflatoxins on rumen function on cellular protein dynamics, and elucidation of tolerance limits for practical feeding. Prof. of Eminence Report, NDRI, Karnal.

Balaraman, N. and Arora, S.P. 1984. Indian J. Anim, Nut, 1 : 65 – 68.

Balaraman, N. and Arora, S.P. 1985. Indian J. Anim, Sci., 56- : 1300-01.

Barrows, S.B.D., Rossi. A.L. and Ngoueria, D.M. 1978. Nutr. Abstr. Revs. (1978) 48: 165.

Bhat, R.V., Nagarajan, V. and Tulpule, P.G. 1978. Health Hazards of Mycotoxins in India. NIN, Hyderabad.

Brekke, O. L., Stringfellow, A.C. and Peplinski, A.J. 1978. J. Agr, Food Chem., 26 : 1383-1389.

Carnaghan, R.B.A. 1965. Nature, 208-308.

Campbell, T. C. and Stoloff, L. 1974. J. Agr. Food Chem. 22 : 1006-1015.

Ciegler. A, Lillehoj, E.B., Peterson, R.E. and Hall, H.H. 1966. Appl. Microbiol, 14 : 934-939.

Dickens, J. W. 1977. J. Am. Oil Chem. Soc. 54 : 225A-228A

Edds, G. T. 1973. J. Am. Vet. Med. Assoc. 163 :304-309.

Fulsounder, A. B. and Shukla, P.C. 1978. Indian J. Anim, Sci., 48 : 145.

Goldblatt, L. A. 1971. J. Am. Oil Chem. Soc., 48 ; 605-610.

Gumbmann, M. R., Williams, S.N., Booth, A.N., Vohra, P., Ernst, R.A. and Bethard, M. 1970. Proc. Soc. Expt. Biol. Med., 134: 683-688.

Kubena, F. and Harvey, R.B. 1988. Egg Industry, p.33

Lee, L. S., Cucullus, A.F. and Poms Jr. W.A. 1977. J. Am, Oil Chem. Soc. 54: 238A-241A

Mathur, C. F., Smith, R.C. and Hawkins, G.E., 1976. J. Dairy Sci., 59: 455-458.

Mishra, R. S. and Singh, R. S. 1978. Current Sci., 47: 396-397.

Newberne, P. M. 1973. J. Am. Vet. Med. Assoc. 13: 1262.

Patel, P.M., Netke, S.P., Gupta, B.S. and Dabadghao, A.K. 1981. Indian J. Anim, Sci. 51: 402-407.

Pier, A. C., 1973. J. Am. Vet. Med, Assoc. 163: 1268-69.

Rao, P. V. 1982. Avian. Res. 66: 110

Rayner, E. T., Koltun, S. P. and Dollear, F. G. 1977. J. Am. Oil Chem. Soc. 54: 142A-144A.

Reddy, D. N. Rao, P. V., Reddy, V. R. and Yadgiri, B. 1984. Indian J. Anim, Sci., 54: 68-73.

Sinha, R. R. P. and Arora, S. P. 1982. Indian J. Nuclear Agric. Biol., 11 : 87-89.

Sinha, R. R. P. and Arora, S. P. 1984. Indian J. Animal Nutr., 1: 19-23.

Sinha, R. R. P. and Arora, S. P. 1985. Indian Anim. Nutr. 2 : 194-196.

Singh, T., Tyagi, R. P. S. and Baburam. 1984. Indian J. Dairy Sci. 37:167-170.

Southern. L. L. and Clawson. A. J. 1979. J. Anim. Sci. 49: 1007-1011,

Shukla, S. K. and Pachauri, S. P. 1985. Indian Vet. J. 62: 341-342.

Tung, H. T., Donaldson, W. E. and Hamilton, P. B. 1972. Toxicol, Appl, Pharmocol., 22 : 97-104.

Valid, J., Dawra, R. K., Sharma, O. P. and Negi, S. S. 1981. Vet. and Human Toxicol., 23 : 436-438.

Wogan, G. N., 1968. Fed. Proc. 27: 932-938.

Wragg, J. B., Ross, V. C. and Legator, M. S. 1967. Proc. Soc. Expt. Biol. Med., 125-: 1052-55.

Yadagiri, B. and Tulpule, P. G. 1974. Indian J. Dairy Sci. 27: 293-297.

CHAPTER 22

MYCOTOXINS: AN OVERVIEW OF THEIR IMPORTANCE, PREVENTION AND CONTROL

Ramesh V Bhat,
National Institute of Nutrition,
Hyderabad 500007

1. INTRODUCTION

Mycotoxins are natural products produced by certain moulds which grow on agricultural commodities under certain conditions. Mycotoxin producing moulds are widely distributed in nature. Agricultural commodites are vulnerable to mould damage during pre as well as post-harvest stages of production. Mould infection of products such as grains, seeds and nuts and toxins produced are often heterogenously distributed especially when stored in bulk. In the case of stored grains that are not sufficiently ventilated moulds starts to develop under conducive environments in pockets of moisture accomulation resulting from difference in temperatures. Although many toxic mould metabolites have been products, so far only a few of them have been found to occur naturally in foods and feed ingredients.

It has long been recognized that foods and feeds contaminated with moulds on consumption may cause serious health problems which could even end in fatalties. For many centuries poisoning due to consumption of bread made from rye infected with ergot has been recognized in Europe. The disease ergotism due to ergot alkaloids has been found to affect men and animals. Alimentary Toxic Alenkia was reported to occur in wintered grains that had been infected with various fungi on the Fusarium spp. However, it is the discovery of aflatoxins, the toxic metabolites of *Aspergillus flavus* and *A. parasiticus* as the causal agent of the turkey X disease which had provided the new impetus for the development of the field of Mycotoxicology. The disease involving death of more than 100,000 turkeys in England following the ingestion of imported groundnut meal contaminated with aflatoxin highlighted health and economic problems of mycotoxin contamination.

Aflatoxin is probably the most studied and widely known mycotoxin. The term aflatoxin is used to refer to a class of chemical of compounds of related structure among which aflatoxin B_1 is the most potent. The high risk commodities for aflatoxin include cereals like maize, parboiled rice, oil seeds like groundnut, cotton seed and certain tree nuts and dried fruits. Aflatoxin contamination may occur at any stage of crop production and marketing. Although the fungus *A. flavus* has been traditionally considered to be a storage mould it has also been found to occur during preharvest conditions. Aflatoxins can be found not only in obviously mouldy foods, but more importantly also in foods which upon visual inspection appear to be suitable for direct human consumption. Aflatoxin can be retained in both cake and oil during extraction of oil from nuts. If mild cattle consume aflatoxin contaminated feed, part of the toxin gets metabolized in the body and secreted in mild as aflatoxin MI.

Contamination by aflatoxin is generally considered to be a problem in tropical and subtropical regions of Asia, Africa and Latin America, where the temperature and humidity conditions are favourable for growth of *Aspergillus flavus*. However, mycotoxins have also been found in temperate countries of Europe and North America thus signifying that mycotoxins are indeed a global problem. The most recent example of serious concern due to aflatoxins was contamination of 25% of the maize crop in USA in 1988 following an unprecedented drought resulting in extensive newspaper coverage, congressional actions and diplocatic upheavals.

2. Importance of Mycotoxins

During the last three decades mycotoxins have been attracting global attention in view of their health, economical and political considerations. Realizing the significance of mycotoxins, national Governments in various countries have been investing on research inputs on several aspects of mycotoxins and initiating administrative action of formulating legislations and implementing regulatory measures in control of mycotoxins.

2.1 Trade and Economic Aspects

Mycotoxins are known to cause significant economic and trade problems at almost every stage of marketing between the producer and ultimate consumers. However, reliable published information on the economic and trade aspects o contamination by mycotoxins is limited when available is not expressed in quantitative terms. The studies and statistics available are often incomplete restricted to aflatoxin only. Hence it is difficult to provide an estimate of economic losses due to mycotoxins. Outright losses of food and feed could be considerably large but not quantifiable at present. Losses of livestock could be spectacular with death of large number of animals but other losses such as lowered meat, egg or poultry productivity, deterioration in quality, poor work performance could be greater in aggregate, though less obvious.

The significance of mycotoxins in the international trade are being increasingly recognized by both the developed and the developing countries. During the last few years the export of agricultural commodities like groundnut, cottonseed, pistachio nuts, copra, and their derivatives, etc. have been affected especially from developing countries, while the export of maize has been affected mainly from the U.S.A. The world volume of the agricultural products like maize, groundnut, copra, palm nuts and oil seed cake and meal which can some of the high risk commodities for aflatoxins is about 100 millions metric tones of which the share of developing countries is over 20 million metric tones. The Indian export of 850 thousand tones of agricultural commodities and their byproducts like groundnut, cottonseed and their derivatives valued at 100 million US$ in 1976 have been reduced to 200 thousand tones valued at 20 million US$ in 1986 due to the problems of aflatoxins (Bhatt 1988). Although countries like India have made up to the problems ofvaluable foreign exchange earnings, by exporting alternate commodities like soyabean extractions which do not have the aflatoxins, in countries like Senegal where groundnut accounts for over 40% of the total national exports the importance of aflatoxins is obvious to the national economy. There were examples of commodities like chillies exported from India being rejected by Japan because of aflatoxins. The export commodities from the region when received attention in the past as having problem of aflatoxin contamination include maize and tapicoca in Thailand, groundnut in Indonesia, palm kernels in Malaysia, copra in Sri Lanka, Philippines and Vanuatu, pistachio nuts in Iran, and almonds in Afghanistan.

Besides the loss of valuable foreign exchange earnings, the cost of inspection, sampling and analysis of aflatxosin during preshipments as well as analysing them again in the important countries is considerable. In India over 10 companies with a chain of 60 laboratories in the private sector over established facilities and are routinely analysing samples exclusively meant for export. Many countries of Asia do not have aflatoxin testing facilities priorto export in their own countries and as such have to depend on reports of analysis carried out at destination of import. Under such circumstances analysis costs will be much more. In addition, the reports will be one-sided and there is no scope to contest the results.

Generally as a consequence of stringent quality specifications, best of the commodities (which are free from aflatoxin) is exported while substandard commodities not acceptable to the foreign buyers are circulated within the country. The economic cost of including such substandard commodities in the diet of animal is substantiated by the recent example of a case of study in a poultry farm in India. As a result of feeding poultry with groundnut cake having 0.7 ppm of aflatoxin the egg production has declined by 27%. A summary calculation of the cost burden over a three-week period including those of reduced egg production, mortality of birds, additional expenditure of an alternate protein sources, medical and analysis expenditure amounted to US$ which is over 10% of the initial investment of the poultry farm.

It has been indirectly estimated that in the U.K. alone the finance losses incurred in poultry industry due to aflatoxins may likely be 500,000 pounds. One well known feed manufaturer is reported to have paid out compensation without commitment totalling 125,000 pounds for the loss of turkeys in 250 the USA 143 millions dollar was lost annually due to consumption of mycotoxin contaminated feed in the broiler industry (Hesseltine 1986).

A new demand that is likely to put forward by the farmers lobby which is now being organized in many of the developing countries of the world is demand towards subsidy cost for the rain-damaged mycotoxin-contaminated crop. During the 1987 season substantial quantities of wheat crop in India was affected by unseasonal rains at the time of harvest and the subsequent growth of the production of trichothecenes. the Central Government of India provided a subsidy of 0.5 US$ per quintal of wheat of the millers to buy the rain-damaged wheat. Likewise in USA if the 1989-90 maize crop fails like that of 1988-89 crop and gets contaminated with aflatoxins there is a congressional move to provide subsidy to the farmer (Caldwell, 1989),

Besides their costs, the loss to the primary producer on account of mould damage and mycotoxin contamination in terms of outright food /feed loss, reduced prices, fetched for contaminated crops, potential loss of outlets, reduced productivity of livestocks leading to less income, are considerable. In addition the traders especially exporters lose income and reputation. The loss of the national exchequer in terms of reduced foreign exchange earnings, increased cost of inspection, sampling, analysis research, surveillance, complicance procedures, training and extension programmes, cost of detoxification and subsidy would also be considerable. In addition trade firictions between exporters and importers as to whether the contamination had occurred before exporting or during voyage in ships had occurred in the past. Also, there were disputes and disagreements between importing and exporting countries on the methodology of sampling, different analytical methodology for estimation of aflatoxins as well as fixation of tolerance limits. The risk of rejection of commodities after they have reached destination in Europe or Japan where there are better facilities for aflatoxin estimation deters the exporters in exporting to these destinations. Countries which do not have stringent quality specifications, countries which agree for barter trade are preferred for export but lesser price is offered and often payments in local currency instead of US$ have to be accepted.

2.2 Health Effects

The harmful effects of mycotoxins on human and animal health have been well recognized. However, vital statistics on mycotoxin-induced diseases are generally lacking. The mycotoxins have been demonstrated to induce adverse effects in laboratory and farm animals. A variety of tissues and organs such as the liver, kidney, nervous and the gastro-intestinal system can be affected depending on the mycotoxin. They may also weaken the immune system of the body. Some of the mycotoxins like aflatoxins have been shown to be mutagenic, carciogenic and teratogenic. Mycotoxins have also been recorded to be responsible for imbalances in feed-live weight conversion ratio in farm animals and lowering their productivity. Besides when mammals ingest aflatoxin contaminated diet the toxin can pass through the milk. Annex 1 summarized the possible harmful effects of some mycotoxins on human/animal health.

So far in the contemporary world evidences for cause and effect relationship hepatitis in India in 1975, in Kenya in 1982 and possible Malaysia in 1988 (the last one yet to be conclusively demonstrated) Entero-ergotism in India in 1976, vascular ergotism in Ethopia in 1979 and deoxynivalenol mycotoxicosis in India in 1989. (Bhatetal 1989 Epidemiological studies have shown an association between dietary aflatoxin exposure and the high incidence of primary liver carcinoma in Philippines, Thailand, Indonesia, Kenya, Swaziland etc. The limiting factors of these studies were that the population intake data were used and no individual intake and other factors such as hepatitis B virus were not considered. Aflatoxin have also been detected in biological samples like blood and urine of children suffering from Kwashiorkor in Sudan and neighboring African countries, from Reyes syndrome in Thiland, USA and from children suffering from childhood cirrhosis in India which indicate the possibility to a role for aflatoxins in the causation or accenturation of the clinical manifestation of these diseases. However, still may gaps exist in our knowledge thus the need for more descriptive and analytical epidemiological studies, which may in turn require better methods in clinical work for detection of mycotoxin in tissues and biological fluids.

3. *Prevention and control of Mycotoxins with special Reference to Aflatoxins*

3.1 Prevention

Recognition of the problems of mycotoxins in various countries calls for appropriate programms for the prevention of control of mycotoxins. These include not only the prevention of mycotoxins formation in agricultural commodities but also their removal through detoxification or decontamination routine surveillance, regulatory measures to control the flow of mycotoxin contaminated commodities in national and international trade as well as information, education and communication drive. All these approaches form part of the strategies to minimize the problems of mycotoxin contamination. However, most of these efforts are limited to aflatoxins.

Prevention of aflatoxin formation in agricultural commodities at farm-levels require better farm management practices including the use of fungus toxin resistant varieties of plants, proper irrigation techniques and fertilizer practices, pest control, crop rotation. Besides high moisture and humidity the factors that favour aflatoxin include high temperature water stress under drought conditions, soil fungal inoculation and extent of insect damage. It is generally recommended that for safe storage, cereal grains should be dried to a moisture content of 13% or less, soybeans, to 12%, groundnuts to 8% and cottonseed to 10%. Safe moisture levels however, vary with the temperature and the time duration at which the commodity is stored. For example aflatoxin concentration can increase approximately 10-fold in a three day period when maize is stored with a higher moisture content. Improving the storage conditions has been one of the important aspect of minimize the aflatoxin formation. Application of chemicals either industrial chemicals like volatile fatty acids or natural aplant extracts help in preventing fungal contamination.

In general blending of contaminated food or feed with good quality produce in order to reduce levels of mycotoxin below the permissible or detectable limit has been practised in the past in many countries. However the risk of adopting such an approach has been highlighted by the Indian experience during 1987 outbreak of deoxynivalenol mycotoxicosis in humans. The rain-affected wheat damaged by moulds was blended with 50% of good wheat by the millers while converting wheat to ordinary and refined wheat flour. But despite such dilution the consumption of these commodities lead to mild form of mycotoxicosis in humans. diverting contaminated commodities as animal feed would also result in diseases in animals or in lowering their productivity in terms of milk or egg yield or deterioration in meat quality,

Recent studies indicate that certain food processing techniques can reduce the aflatoxin levels but generally it is believed that traditional processes such as heating, roasting, baking etc. does not always completely eliminate the toxins.

3.2 Detoxification

In order to avoid complete loss of contaminated products, methods for detoxifying feed products have been evolved. Such products for the use by animals only. The various detoxification techniques can be classified as follows:

- Extraction of aflatoxins by solvents
- Inactivation of toxins by physical (heat, cooking, roasting) chemical or biological means.

One of the most promising methods of detoxification of aflatoxin contaminated products had been the approach of ammonia detoxification, which after two decades of extensive study has been established in pilot plant scale in USA, UK, India and commercially practised in Senegal. Such a process of ammoniation of groundnut cake is feasible on a large scale up to 800 tones capacity designed miniplans (Overseas Development Natural Resources Institute of England) as is being envisaged in India. The major reason why several developing countries are reluctant tomake heavy investments in such plants is the reluctance of EEC buyers to guarantee the purchase of detoxified meal in the absence of a clear policy directive on the part of the EEC food and feed regulatory authorities. A fear has been expressed in certain quarters that the ammonia detoxified groundnut meal if ingested by the animals may again be reconverted in the stomach of the animals to parent toxic compound. Until such doubts are clarified and necessary clearance for allowing the use of detoxified groundnut mean in EEC markets, the process of detoxification is unlike to gain momentum. However, despite these limitations, it must be admitted that the starting of such detoxification units will certainly help the developing countries in distributing the detoxified products in the domestic market, itself. Preliminary enquiries with the users of groundnut cake like the poultry farmers in India have indicated that they are willing to pay the premium to cover the detoxification cost for the groundnut meal. Thus, one detoxified cake have a new image to give confidence in their safety, the higher cost of 10% for producing detoxified groundnut meal which has been considered as a limiting factor in the highly competitive market could be overcome by the fact that the protein value of the detoxified meal is higher than the original meal.

3.3 Decontamination or Segregation approach

A practical solution of the problem of aflatoxin is groundnuts that has been experimented in three countries viz; Australia, the USA and Malawi, is the process of selected seggregation and sorting and then removing aflatoxin-contaminated kernels. In Malawi the Agricultural Development and Marketing corporation purchases shelled groundnuts from small farmers, electronically sorts, and tests the nuts for aflatoxins at the groundnut factors. The process of handshelling and hand grading of groundnuts by the small farmers followed by regarding and aflatoxin testing of the nuts has earned Malwi a reputation as a source of high quality of the nuts from the confectionary trade. In the USA the National Peanut Council has initiated a peanut quality enhancement project to explore the concept of screening farmers stock of groundnut prior to marketing as an appropriate and economically-viable approach to quality enhancement. The farmers' stock of groundnuts is screened with a belt screen, which separated it into two, sizes i.e. groundnuts, which ride screen of particular size and those, which fall through these screens. The nuts are then graded, cleaned, shelled, sorted and the aflatoxin content is analysed. Such belt screening procedures are reported to be useful in reducing aflatoxin levels in groundnuts. The Queensland Department of Primary Industries at Kingaroy is following similar approach for the decontamination by segregation in Australia. An operation research product on the above pattern is under consideration in India.

3.4 Regulatory Control of Mycotoxins

Regulatory control measures on mycotoxins especially aflatoxins had been initiated by several countries in order to protect the public health and to promote trade at national and international levels. These standards include limits or tolerance levels, sampling and analytical methodologies. Specific mycotoxin legislation has been developed mostly for aflatoxins, but a few countries like India have proposed regulation in addition to other mycotoxins like ergot alkaloids and deoxynivalenol. There is lack of uniformity in the limits fixed in various countries and international harmonization efforts are under progress. Generally, the countries, which have basic interest in the export of agricultural commodities, prefer a stringent limit. Some of the countries are fixing the limits based on economic compulsions, other on analytical capabilities to detect minimum quantities. Often criticism is levelled against such practices since they do not take into account the possible errors in sampling and analyses variabiolities. It should also be recognized that certain classes of food are consumed in relatively small quantities (e.g. red pepper) for which the general application is restrictive. Consumer groups in countries like the USA had in the recent past resorted to legal action demanding the regulatory authorities to firmly establish tolerance limits for mycotoxins rather than use discretionary powers in regulating mycotoxins with action levels. Such actions had led to the possibility to a bill being introduced in the US house to require an USDA to set standards for aflatoxin testing and to require federal grain inspectors to screen export-bound US maize.

In their directive on the fixing of maximum permitted levels for undesirable substances and products in feeding stuffs the European community has differentiated the permissible levels for aflatoxin B_1 on the basis of intended use i.e. straight feeding stuffs, complete feeding stuffs and complementary feeding stuffs (See Annex 1) It was considered necessary not only to limit the presence of aflatoxin to an acceptable level but also reverve the contaminated raw materials to recognized manufactures of compound feedstuffs in order to ensure that the necessary dilutions are performed to guarantee compliance with the maximum permitted levels laid down in the directive for feeding stuffs. The product would have to be accompanied by documents bearing the words 'reserved exclusively for recognized manufactures" of compound feeding stuffs, not to be fed unprocessed to livestock and indicating the content of aflatoxins. Recently initiative had been taken in countries like the Netherlands and Switzerland to set maximum levels for aflatoxin M_1 in milk and milk products which again has an effect on permissible limit for aflatoxin in complementary feed in cattle.

In India, a risk assessment study was attempted for fixing tolerance limits for deoxynivalenol (DON). The actual level of DON mycotoxin responsible for causing disease outbreak in humans based on the actual food consumption data was obtained through diet survey and laboratory analysis. The data was further corroborated by similar data calculated on the basis of natural outbreaks of deoxynivalenol mycotoxicosis in farm animals as well as result of experimental studies in pups and primates. Based on these findings, a tolerance level of 34 ppb of deoxynivalenol in wheat was suggested. The limit is more stringent that the limits of 1000 ppb of DON in wheat suggested in Canada and USSR and recommended in USA for voluntary compliance but more liberal than 5 ppb limit fixed in Romania.

The stringent levels of mycotoxin regulation enforced by importing countries put heavy burdens on international food trade. The income of some of the developing countries whose income depend on the export of food products susceptible to mycotoxin contamination suffered difficulties in trade because of differences among country regulations and food rejections on the basis of compliance of strict regulations. Action is needed for proposing international levels of mycotoxins as soon as possible in order to control those difficulties.

PROPOSED GUIDELINE LEVELS FOR AFLATOXINS FOR VARIOUS ANIMAL FEEDSTUFFS AS ESTABLISHED BY THE EEC

Straight feeding stuffs	50 mg/kg (B_1)
Complete feeding stuffs for cattle, sheep and goats (except dairy cattle, calves and lambs)	50 mg/kg (B_1)
Complete feeding stuffs for the pigs and poultry (except young animals)	20 mg/kg (B1)
Other complete feeding stuffs	10 mg/kg (B_1)
Supplementary feeding stuffs for cattle, sheep and goats (except dairy animals, calves and lambs)	50 mg/kg (B_1)
Supplementary feeding stuffs for pigs and poultry (except young animals)	30 mg/kg (B_1)
Other supplementary feeding stuffs	10 mg/kg (B_1)
Groundnut, copra, palm kernel, cottonseed, babassu, maize and products derived from the processing thereof	200 mg/kg (B_1)

REFERENCES

1. Austwick K.C.P. In Mycotixic Fungi, Mycotoxins, Mycotoxicosis: An Encyclopaedic Handbook (Eds.) Wyllie T. D. and Morehouse L. G., Marcell Dekker Inc. New York Vol. II 279-301, 1978.
2. Bhat R.V. Mould Deterioration in Agricultural commodities During Transit, . Microbiol. 7: 219-225, 1988.
3. Bulatao-Jayme, J., Almero, E.M., Castor C.A., Jardeleze T.R. and Salamat L.A. Int. J. Epidemio 11 : 112, 1982.
4. Caldell E.F. Cereal Industry Newsletter, Cereal Foods Worlds 34: 573, 1989.
5. Carnevale, C. 1987, Food Contaminants- FDAs Concern. Cereal Foods World 32: 812-815, 1987.
6. Hesseltine, C.V. Global Significance of Mycotoxins in Bioactive Molecules-Mycotoxins and Phycotoxins Eds Steyn P.S. and Vleggaar R. Elsevier Amsterdam 1-9, 1986.
7 Rao B.S., Rao V.S. Ramakrishna, V. and Bhat R.V. Rapid and Specific

and Method for Screening Ergosterol an Index of Fungal Contamination in Cereal Grains, Food Chem. 31: 51-56, 1989.

8. Sushidhar R.B. Bhat, R.V. and Vasanthi S. Rapid Detection of Aflatoxin by Pressure vinculum Technique: A Collaboratie Trail. Curr. Sci. 58: 882-884, 1989.
9. Waibel. J. In Stickprogengrosse fur die Bestimmung von Aflatoxin in Erdnusse. Deutsche Lebensmittel-rundschau 73: 553-593, 1972.
10. Whitaker, T.B. and Dickens, J.W. The Negative Binomial Distribution J. Am. Oil Chem Soc. 49: 590-593, 1972.
11. Bhat, R.V. Sashidhar R.B. Ramakrishna Y and K.L. Munshi outbreak of Trichthecene mycotoxicosis associated with consumption of mould damaged wheat products in Kashmir Valley, India Lancei i : 35-37, 1989.

CHAPTER

23

FACTORS AFFECTING TOXIN PRODUCTON BY FUNGI AND ITS CONTROL

Annapuran Jetty
Scientist Indian Institute of Chemical Technology, Hyderabad - 500 007.

Mycotoxic fungi and their resulting threat to food and feed stuffs worldwide continue to have an extensive impact on the welfare on human and animal populations. Since early times these fungi have made their mark, but only lately have we been able to appreciate the extent of their impact. For many centuries, poisoning due to the consumption of rye infected with the parasitic fungus ergot (*Claviceps purpurea)* has been recognised. The toxins, the ergot alkaloids produced by this fungus, were identified over 100 years ago and caused death and an enormous degree of suffering to many people and animals.

However, it was not until 1961 that mycotoxins, that in particular aflatoxins, were recognised as presenting real and urgent problems in the sectors of humans and animal health. The term aflatoxin referes to a group of secondary fungal metabolites that are potent animal toxins and carcinogens. Chemically, aflatoxins are highly substituted coumarisn. They are because they are first isolated from the fungus *A. flavus*. The range of foodstuffs potentially affected by mycotoxic fungi and the numbers of microbial species has been extensively increased in recent years. Although the expidemic occurrences seem to have lessened, the endemic and subtler effects so less destructive appear to be increasing.

It is, therefore, clear that mycotoxin contamination of foods and feeds is a world problem, and it would be useful to review in detail, the factors, which might in one way or another influence the fungi or mycotoxin development.

The growth of mould and the production of aflatoxin on/in various agricultural commodities depends upon several factors such as fungal substrate, moisture, relative humidity, temperature, time, growth and maturity and storage conditions etc. The environmental conditions under which the agricultural commodities are harvested, transported, handled, stored and marketed will, to a great extent, determine the extent of contamination of aflatoxin in these commodities.

Aflatoxins are largely produced by fungi belonging to *A. flavus* group which includes *A. flavus, A parasiticus, A. oryae* and *A. tamari.* Other species of fungi belonging to *Aspergilus* and *Penicillus* also produce aflatoxin. *A. flavus* can also grow and produce different types of aflatoxin on several foods and feedstuffs. Aflatoxin B_1, B_2, G_1 and G_2 are the major aflatoxins. However all agricultural commodities do not support aflatoxin production equally. Cereal grains, in general appear to be good substrates for toxin production than oil seeds. This may be due to high proportion of carbohydrates in cereals which may be metabolised by fungi more easily than facts. However, more incidences of aflatoxins production in oilseeds like groundnuts and cotton seeds are reported probably because of favourable environmental conditions. Moisture and relative humidity are the most important factors in mould growth and aflatoxin production. The safe storage mositure in equilibrium with 70 per cent relative humidity. *A.flavus* is a mesophilic fungus and has minimum, optimum and maximum growth temperature of 6-8°C, 36-38°C and 44-46°C, respectively. These values may be influenced by other growth conditions such as aeration, moisture, nutrients etc. Optimum temperature for growth of fungus may be optimum for production of aflatoxin. Aflatoxins are produced in the range of 20 to 35°C temperatures on various agricultural commdities. The optimum time for aflatoxin production varies with temperature. The time for aflatoxin production on different agricultural commodities has been reported from 2-13 days at different temperatures.

Old pods and kernels of groundnuts were invaded by *A. flavus* than freshly dog immature and mature pods and kernels. Mechanical damage to kernels/grains or pods or nuts during harvest, handling or storage or cracking during heat drying can increase their vulnerability of fungi. Damage to kernels/grains also increases the nutrient the kernels/grains and act the as vectors for fungal transmission. Fungi are highly aerobic organisms. However, their requirements of oxygen for vegetative growth, sporulation and spore germination are highly variable. The production of aflatoxin is inversely related to the concentrations of CO_2 and O_2. Irradiation has been suggested as a means of increasing storage life of agricultural commodities. But it also increases the susceptibility of product to storage fungi especially *Aspergillus* sp. which leads to aflatoxin formation.

Some varieties of field crops are relatively resistant to fungal development and subsequently aflatoxin formation. The development of commercially popular varieties that would resist the development of toxigenic mould under bad conditions of storage or that would completely inhibit the elaboration of the toxin would due an ideal solution to save from aflatoxin.

A. flavus is frequency associated with numerous other microorganisms, particularly with stored grains. Microbial competition between fungi for substrate under favourable environmental conditions will reduce or restrict the amount of aflatoxin formation. *A flavus* or competing microorganisms might absorb aflatoxin following its formation in the substrate. Processing of some agricultural commodities to make these edible may reduce aflatoxin content in the final product. Environmental conditions, drought condition, insect attract of standing crops, wind velocity and irrigation may affect the aflaotoxin contents of different crops. Plant protection chemicals like insecticides and fungicides have decreasing effect on aflatoxin production. Number of chemical compounds have inhibitory effect against aflatoxin production. Majority of species and plant extracts also have inhibitory effects on aflatoxin production. Some of the trace elements have been shown to be necessary for aflatoxin production.

In part, this results from the awareness brought about the document cause and effect relationship. A wealth of knowledge about mycotoxic fungi, their toxins and the resulting toxicosis has been demonstrated in scientific literature throughout the world.

Measure for prevention of contamination of detoxification

Generally the presence of mould in foods and feeds has been recognised as undesirable. Aflatoxins in many food stuffs have been demonstrated to cause sickness and death in farm animals and human beings. At lower levels they may not cause overt signs of illumes but can cause reduced growth rate in youngsters, lowered feed efficiency, reduced egg production in poultry and lowered resistance to infectious diseases. Hence, it is very necessary to reduce the level of aflatoxin in food and feeds or to remove aflatoxin completely from them.

1. *Prevention of aflatoxin contamination*

The prevention of aflatoxin formation on agricultural commodities is fundamentally a problem of curtailing fungal growth. Mould contamination can occur on crop during crop development, harvesting and drying, storage, transport, processing etc.

(a) Prevention before harvest: To ensure a mould-free product at harvest, farmers must utilize proper agronomic techniques during planting and cultivation that will provide conditions for optimum crop development.

1. Agronomic practices: crop rotation, proper irrigation
2. Use of resistant varieties of seeds
3. Pesticides and chemicals to control mould

(b) During harvesting and drying:

1. Prevention of mechanical injury
2. Harvesting of crops at full maturity
3. Proper drying

(c) During storage

1. Insect control during storage
2. Adequate aeration

(d) During transport

1. Disinfections of transport containers
2. Use of tarpaulins, air-tight container to avoid moisture absorption during shipment

(e) During processing

1. Protection of crops during processing from any conditions encouraging growth of fungi
2. Segregation of damaged portion of crop by physical means
3. Inactivation of aflatoxin by methods which will not result in new toxic substances into the feed.

II. Decontamination

1. Physical removal of contaminated kernels or nuts

III. Detoxification

It refers to the techniques which remove the toxin from or within the unit or kernel or destroy or inactivate the toxin from the product.

A detoxification process must be technical and economically-viable and must meet the following criteria:

1. It must destroy or inactivate the aflatoxin
2. It should not produce or leave toxic or carcinogenic residues in the final product.
3. It must destroy fungal spores and mycelia which could under favourable conditions proliferate and form new toxins
4. It must preserve the nutritive value and acceptibility of the product.
5. It should not significantly alter important technological properties.

(a) Removal of aflatoxin
   1. Physical removal (Absorption)
   2. Chemical means (Solvent separation)
   3. Processing
   4. Irradiation

(b) Inactivation of aflatoxin
   1. Physical methods
   2. Autoclaving
   3. Cooking
   4. Roasting
   5. Light

IV. Microbiological means

Use of other microbes to detoxify mycotoxins

There treatments may add some cost to the product. However, such treatment may permit us to make use of the contaminated foods and feeds which otherwise have to be destroyed or rejected.

REFERENCES

Mycotoxins in Food Stuff, G.N. Wagan, ed. MIT Press, Cambridge, Massachusetts.

FAO Food and Nutrition Paper. Conference Report on Mycotoxins eld in Nairobi, 19-27. Food and Agriculture Organization of United Nations, Rome, 1977.

Salunkhe, D.K., R.N., Adsule and D.N. Padule (Eds.) Aflatoxins in Food and Feeds, 1987. Metropolitan, New Delhi - 110 064.

CHAPTER 24

THE ROLE OF AFLATOXIN IN HUMAN HEALTH

Dr. S. M. Mohiuddin,
Associate Professor and Head, Department of Pathology, CVSs,
Rajendranagar, Hydrabad - 500030.

Disease caused by moulds and mycotoxin in farm animals and human beings have been realized long back, however, it is neglected, with an exception to Ergotism. Ergotism is a best known disease caused by mycotoxins in Europe during middle ages, when the outbreaks of apparent madness were attributed to a diabolic possession.

Pencillium spp. was experimental shown to be associated with nervous disorders (Miyake *et al.*,1940). "Yellow rice" toxicity in Japan has been traced to contamination with fungi *Pencillium islandieum* during the early century (Uragewehi *et al.*,1961). In Russia, outbreaks of mycotoxicosis, causing alimentary toxin aleukia (ATA) was recorded during the World War II (Jotte, 1966).

Since the outbreak of Turkey "X' disease in Great Britain, during the 1960s, a worldwide attention has been attached to diseases caused by mycotoxins. This disease is caused by aflatoxins, are produced by fungus *Aspergillus flavus* and *Parasiticus* and have been reported from all parts of the world. Aflatoxin production been reported from all parts of the world. Aflatoxin production fungal strains are a widely distributed in air and soil and are capable to grow on a variety of natural substances apart from groundnut. It has been reported from rice, corn, soybeans, oats, wheat and mutton. They produce aflatoxin B_1, B_2, G_1 and G_2, of the B_1 is highly toxic than others. The metabolics of the toxin are demonstrated in milk, meat and eggs (Shank *et al.*,1971b).

Since human experiments are impossible efforts have been taken in different parts of the world to correlate the effects of aflatoxin, its metabolites on human health. It is mostly based on epidemiological observations, outbreak, supported by analytical data of the toxin levels. However, there is no direct evidence implicating aflatoxin as the cause of disease.

Effect in children

There is volumenous information and data on the toxicological action of mycotoxin including aflatoxin in various animal species. However, there is paucity of direct information on the degree of susceptibility of man to aflatoxin. Hence, the suggestive evidence derived from animal experiments provide a convincing explanation that the aflatoxins are also effective in humans. Two deaths in children were reported and in both the cases the food they consumed contained aflatoxin (Bowrgeius *et al.,* 1971). Sublethal toxicity due to aflatoxin (0.5-1.0 ug/kg) was reported when Kawshioskor children were fed with peanut meal as a source of protein (Payet *et al.,* 1966). Indian Childhood Cirrhosis (CC) in Indian children is attributed to the aflatoxin, through breast milk, and dietary items such as unrefined oil, parboiled rice (Amla *et al.,* 1969). Twenty children have been reported to suffer, when treated for ICC by dietary supplementation with peanut meal at CFTRI. Mysore, which contained aflatoxin B_1 at 0.3 ug/kg (Amta *et al.,* 1970, 1971). Breast milk was also found to contain aflatoxin B1 in finding corroborated by a similar study in Bangalore (Robinson, 1967).

Several hundred children in the age group of 1-13 years were reported to have diet at Thailand annually of a disease involving acute encephalopally and fatty degeneration of the viscera (EFDV) (Shank *et al.,* 1971a), similar in detail symptom to autopsy specimens from 23 children revealed aflatoxin B_1. A pathology closely resembling EFDV in children was experimentally produced in cynomolgus monkeys on feeding a single dose of aflatoxin B_1 at 13.5 mg/kg body weight. (Bowrgiois *et al.,*1971). In a series of study carried out in Sudan, Nigeria, Ghana and South Africa in both autopsied as well as biopsied lives from children suffering from Kwashiarkar and marasnic Kwasharkar, aflatoxin in range from 62 to 33206 ug/kg were detected (Cutler *et al.,* 1986: Hendrickse, 1984). The major source of aflatoxin among population are groundnuts and peanuts (Hendrickse *et al.,* 1982) and aflatoxin M_1 and M_2 were frequently detected in breast milk of Sudanese women (Culture *et al.,* 1984).

Acute effects

Outbreaks of the aflatoxicosis in man has been reported from Asia and Africa due to eating aflatoxin-contaminated food. Hepatitis caused by eating heavily aflatoxin-contaminated feed was reported in certain tribal communities of India during 1975 and in Kenya during

1981 (Krishnamachari *et al.*, 1975: Naginder *et al.*, 1982). Respiratory symptoms, burning of eyes, nose and throat, fever and chill were noticed in persons engaged to clean moldy grain stores house (Emanuel *et al.*, 1975) and these fungi are identified as *Aspergillus* (Palmgren, 1985).

Neoplastic effects

The etiology of aflatoxicosis and hepatocelular carcinoma in Bantus provides a considerable presumptive evidence that aflatoxin are the major cause rather than hereditary or ethnic origin outbreaks of aflatoxicosis *et al.*,(1982) in Kenya is sufficient proof to document that aflatoxin do have an influence in the aetiology.

Aflatoxin has produced changes in the hereditary material of human cells grow in tissues cultures: which could turn normal into concerns one. The toxin also causes birth defects if it was fed during pregnancy (Legator, 1985). Alveolar cell aurcinoma was noticed in the lungs of a chemical engineer and his colleagues who are looking after the sterilization of Brazilian groundnut meal contaminated with *Aspergillus flavus.* Aflatoxin B1 was detected in the lung tissues (Dvorackova, 1976). In Czechoslovakia, three cases of pulmonary intertitial fibrosis was noticed, who were agricultural workers (Dvorachkova and Pichova, 1986). Various types of respiratory tract cancer was noticed in a Dutch groundnut oil factory workers exposed to 0.039-2.5 ug/kg aflatoxin (Van Niew Wenhuze *et al.*, 1973). The cause and effect relation of the incidence of hepatoma due to aflatoxin has been well documented by Campbell and Stoloff (1984). A positive correlation between Hepato cellular carcinoma (HCC) and aflatoxin ingestion by man has been established from the studies carried out in Kenya, Swaziland, the Transkei region of South Africa, Mozambique and Thailand (Bhat, 1989).

A global survey carried out at different parts of the world showed that maize groundnut are the commodities mostly affected by florin (Hessetine, 1986). In the developed countries like the USA, the survey showed that the level of aflatoxin is five times higher in maize than groundnut (Stoloff, 1985).

It is recognized that when animals consumed aflatoxin contained feed, is metabolised in the body and may enter milk as aflatoxin M_1 and M_2 or may be found in meat and egg which are consumed by man. The level of the metabolites that are present in these products are, however, lower than those in agricultural products. However, aflatoxin M_1 and M_2 from the earlier studies has been reported to be responsible for the ICC in children. The evidence on acute and chronic diseases in man is lacking due to the consumption of meat and eggs. However, to minimize the health hazard, legislation have been passed in several countries restricting the level of aflatoxin in animal feeds.

Based on these data it is necessary to have more epidemiological studies to further confirm the action of aflatoxin in man. It can also be concluded that evidence, to directly implicate aflatoxin consumption through groundnut and its product, maize and milk is conculsive, but needs further studies in relation to other products like meat and eggs.

REFERENCES

Miyake, I., Na to H., and Tswnoda, H. 1940. Beikoku, Riyo, Kenkyuto, Hokou. 1: 1.

Uraguchi, K., Tatswano, T., Sakei, F.T., Sukioka, M., Sakai, Y., Yonmits, T. and Isaiko, T. 1961. Japan J. Exp. Md. 31: 1.

OHe, A.Z. 1966. Mycotoxin in food stuffs (Wogen, Edt.) p. 77. MI.T. Press, Cambridge, Massachesette.

Cowrgriosis, H. Shank, R.C., Brossman, R.S., Johnson, D., Orwooding, W.L. and Chandavimol, P. 1971. Lab. Invest. 24: 206.

Ayet, M., Cros, J., Qwenurrs, Snakale, M. and Monlanier, M. 1966. Press, Med. 74(13): 649-651.

Nla, I., Kamala, C.S., Gopalarishnal, G.S., Jayaraj, A.P., Screenivasa Murthy, V. and Parpia, H.A.B. 1971. Amer, J. Clin, Nutr. 24: 609.

la, I., Narayan, J.V, Jayaraj, A.P., Sreenivasamurthy, V. and Parpia, H.A.B. 1969. Ind.pased. 6 : 305.

Binson, P. 1967. Clin. Pedia. 610: 57-305,

Ank, R.C., Bowrgiois, C.H., Keschamras, N., and Chnadavimol., P. 1971a. Food Cosmet. Toxicol. 9 : 501

Shnamachari, K.V.A.R., Bhatt, R.V., Nagarajan, V. and Tilka, T.B. 1975. Hepatotoxocity due to aflatoxicosi. An outbreak in Western of India, Lancet 1 : 1061-1063.

Indu, A., Johnson, B.K. Kenya, P.R., Nqura, J.A. Ooheng, D.M., Nanda, H., Omandi, T.N., Jansen, A.J., Ngase, W., Kaviti, acute hepatitis caused by aflatoxin poisoning in Kenya. 1 : 1346-1348.

Aule,. D.A., Wenzel, F.J. and Lowton, B.R. 1975. Pulmonary

Palmgren, M.S. 1985. Microbial and toxin constituents of green dust and their health implication. p. 47-57. In Trichottecenes and other mycotoxins (Lacey, J. ed., Chichester, U.K. Wiley).

Dvorackova, I. 1976. Aflatoxin inhalation and alveolar cell carcinoma. Brit. Med. J. 1 : 691.

Dvorackova, I. Pichova, V. 1986. Pulmonary intestinal fibroiis with evidence of aflatoxin B1 in lung tissue. J. Toxiqtnvir Health, 18 : 153-157.

Van Niew Wenheize, J.P., Herber, R.F.M., Debruin, A., Meyer, I.P.B. and Diba, W.C. 1973. Tijadschrift voor Diergneek 51: 754.

Campbell and Stoloff. 1974.

Bhatt, R.V. 1987. Aflatoxin contamination of groundnut; proceedings of the International workshop, 6-9 Oct. ICRISAT, A.P., India.

Coutler, J.B.S., Suliman, G.I., Lamplwgh, S.M., Mukhtar, B.J. and Hendrickse, R.G. 1986. Amer, Jr. Trop. Med. & Hygi. 35: 360-365.

Hendrickse, R.G. 1984. Transaction of Roy. Soc. Trop. Medi. & Hygi. 78: 427-435.

Hendrickse, R.G. Coulter, J.B.S., Lamplwgh, S.M., Macfarlane, S.B.J., Williams T.E., Omer, M.I.A. and Saliman, G.I. 1982. Brit, Med, Jour. 285: 843-846.

Coulter, J.B.S. Lamphleugh, S.M., Suliman, G.I., Omer, M.I.A. and Hendrickse, R. G. 1984. Annals of Trop. Pedia. 4 : 61-66.

Hesselline, C.N. 1986. Mycotoxins and plytotoxins (Steyn, P.S. and Vleggas R. eds.). Amsterdam. Netherland Elsevier pp. 1-16.

Stoloff, C. 1985. In mycotoxin and plytotoxins (Steyn, P.S. and; vleggaar, R. eds.). Amsterdams, Netherlands, Elsevier, pp. 457-471.

CHAPTER 25

SIMPLE METHODS OF AFLATOXINS DETECTION

S. Vasanthi
National Institute of Nutrition
Hyderabad - 500 007.

INTRODUCTION

The aflatoxins are a group of secondary metabolies produced by the fungi, *Aspergillus flavus* and *Aspergillus parasiticus.* They have been demonstrated to be the most potent hepatocarcinogens in a number of experimental animals and have been associated with a high incidence of human liver cancer in certain parts of the world. Because of their natural occurrence in a wide variety of agricultural commodities, various analytical methods have been developed so that the level of aflatoxin contamination in foods and feeds may be monitored with reasonable accuracy (9,3). Analytical approaches to detection of aflatoxin in foods and feeds mainly involved chemical methods as they are most specific, rapid, and reproducible and possess lower limits of detection than biological methods. The most widely used chemical methods are based on chromatographic techniques like thin layer chromatography (TLC) and High Pressure Lipuid Chromatography (HPLC) and immunoassays like the Radioimmunoassay (RIA) and the Enzyme linked immuno Sorbet Assay (ELISA). These methods are used for screening quantitation and confirmation of aflatoxins, depending on the limits of detection and precision and accuracy required.

Chromatographic techniques

ILC, either visual or denitome trick, is the most frequently used technique for screening and quantitation of aflatoxins, having a limit of detection of 1-0.5 mg (5). HPLC is more sensitive and and rapid and is used mainly for quantitation of aflatoxins. Both the methods involve the basic steps in chromatogorphic analysis, namely, extraction, clean up separation, detection confirmation and quantitation. TLC is advantageous as a screening and quantitation method as more simple extracts can be spotted per plate in the screening test, since only a few standards are needed and the concentration of positive can be estimated in the screening test. HPLC is more rapid and sensitive than TLC as more number of samples of estimated of the first minicolumn by Holaday in 1968, many minicolumns were developed and tested for aflatoxin in a number of agricultural commodities (2). Currently, the Romer's all purpose minicolumn and Holaday Velasco/s minicolumns are used for detection of aflatoxin in foods and feeds and are official procedures of the AOAC (3,4). The major uses of the minicolum techniques are (a) as a rapid screening method in the field or commodity purchasing station to detect the presence or absence of aflatoxin so as to reject or accept a commodity lot and (b) at a Central laboratory to reduce the time needed to test samples that do not contain a detectable amount of aflatoxin.

The principle behind the minicolum technique is similar to that of TLC in that the toxin if first separated from the sample matrix and then detected while still on the minicolumn. The difference lies primarily in the way the sample extract is applied to the minicolumn. In normal TLC methods, a portion of the sample extract is evaporated to dryness, dissolved in a small amount of solvent and portion of the solvent applied to the TLC plate with the help of a microsyringe. In the minicolumn method, a large volume of the extract (1-2 ml) is directly applied to the minicolumn and aflatoxin is detected as a compact blue flocrescent band when viewed under long range UV light.

In India, recently, a simple, rapid, economical, reliable and practically feasible method, namely the Pressure Minicolumn has been developed and collaboratively tested (6, 8).

The Pressure Minicolumn (PMC)

This technique employs commonly available glass syringes, which are tightly packed with certain absorbents. The syringes also allow application of positive pressure which helps in better separation of aflatoxins. The presence of aflatoxins is observed as a compact bluish fluorescent blood under long range UV light. The PMC has been an added advantage of extending the within a relatively short period. However, the use of these methods as rapid screening procedures in safety monitoring programmers is somewhat limited owing to their requirement of expensive and elaborate laboratory facilities, highly trained personnel, & TLC methods of more time-consuming and require extensive sample clean up and expensive solvents.

Immunossay methods

In recent years, immunoassay methods like RIA and ELISA are gaining wider application in aflatoxin detection methodology, as they are rapid, highly sensitive, specific and simple to operate requiring little sample clean up (7). The immunoassay are based on the molecular recognition properties of antibodies. The technique involves interaction between native antigens (like aflatoxin) and specific antibodies leading to precipitation of the antigen-antibody complex which is a measure for the antigen or antibody concentration. Many commercial ELISA kits are currently available. These include Agriscreen, Afla-20, E2-screen, which have been adopted as AOAC Official Its Action procedures for screening aflatoxins in various agricultural commodities and feeds. But the use of these methods is limited in developing culture as they are not easily accessible and are economically prohibitive. Moreover, the enzymes are sensitive to humid conditions and temperature extremes.

Simple methods of aflatoxin detection

Attention is currently focused on the development of simple techniques that are rapid, sensitive, reasonably accurate, inexpensive, requiring little technical expertise and more practically applied such as in the field, farm commodity purchasing stations and public health agencies for surveillance.

The need for such simple and rapid methods for aflatoxin detection prompted the development of minicolumn chromatography. After the development confirmatory tests of aflatoxins on TLC to the minicolumn.

Methods

Reparation of the minicolumn

5 ml glass syringes of borosilicate glass (11 mm i.d.; 9 cm length) are packed with the following adsorbents; a disc of filter paper (Whatman No. 1) the bottom, finely powdered anhydrous sodium sulfate (3 ml), silica gel 60-120 mesh, 5 mm), florisil 100-200 mesh (1 mm), filter paper disc, anhydrous sodium sulfate (4 mm), followed by filter paper disc at the top. Such layer is tightly packed using a plunger of diameter smaller than that of the syringe. The column is activated at 110°C for 1-2 h.

Reparation of the simple

The PMC method has been tested with naturally-contaminated and spiked amples of cereals like rice, wheat, maize and sorghum; oilseeds like peanuts, deoiled peanut cake, deoiled cottonseed cake and animal feeds like poultry feeds (6).

Extraction

Aflatoxins from samples of cereals are extracted by the method of the Barabalok *et al* (1) slightly modifying the procedure by the use of 20% lead cetates for removing interfering compounds instead of ammoniam sulfate (40%). Aflatoxins from oilseeds are extracted by the Best Foods method (9). Poultry seed samples are first subjected to Best Foods methods and then extracted by the Barabalok method.

The step-wise extraction of aflatoxins from naturally-contaminated maize is given below:

Step 1: Shake 10 g sample + 50 ml acetone: water (85:15 v/v) + 2.5 g celite 30 minutes on a wrist arm shaker.

Step 2: Filter the extract through Whatman No.1 filter paper Take 10 ml of the filtrate in a test tube, add 10 ml of 20% feed acetane solution (w/v), mix vigorously for 3-4 minutes and filter through Whatman No. 1 filter paper into a 60 ml separator funnel.

Step 3: Add 2 ml benzene to the filtrate in the separatory funnel and mix thoroughly to extract aflatoxins into the benzene layer.

Step 4 : After phase separation discard the lower layer and collect the upper benzene layer in a test tube containing 400 mg of neutral alumina (active). Mix the contents for 2 minutes on a vortex shaker and allow to stand.

Step 5: Take on millilitre of clean benzene layer from step 4 and slowly load to the activated pressure minicolumn,and allow the layer to enter the column by gravity. Add 3 ml of cleaning solvent (hexane chloroform tetrahydrofuran, 7:2:1) and rapidly drain the solvent by applying pressure with the plunger.

Step 6: Observe the PMC under long range UV high (365 ml) for the presence of a compact blue fluorescent band at the interface of florisil and silica gel. Compare the fluorescene with the fluorescence of standard aflatoxin B1 prepared in a similar way by the PMC technique. By visual comparison of sample fluorescence with standard fluorescence, the sample can be screened as positive or negative for aflatoxin.

Confirmatory tests

After observing the blue fluorescent band of aflatoxin under UV light, keep the column in the hot air oven at 100°C for 5 minutes, to facilitate easy removal of the plunger. Allow the column to come to room temperature. The confirmatory test consists of treatment of the column with one millilitre of trifluoroacetic acid + 20% sulfuric acid in the ratio of 1:1 (v/v) reagent. When viewed under UV light, the treatment gives greenish to blue fluorescence to aflatoxins, indicating their positive presence.

Limits of detection

The limits of detection of the PMC technique for the various agricultural commodities tastes ranges from 25-30 ppb (ng/g) which is the Indian tolerance limit set by the PFA.

Quantitation of aflatoxins by the PMC method

By comparing the intensity of the fluorescent band of the sample with that of the standard, a semi-quantitation of aflatoxins can be achieved using the following equation:

where,

S_2 - Standard aflatoxin concentration method with the fluorescence of the sample.

S_2= Concentration of sample fluorescence methed with standard aflatoxin fluorescence.

V_1 = Volume of the standard of aflatoxin loaded on the column (ml).

V_2 = Volume of sample loaded on the column (ml).

Advantages of the PMC method

1. Size of the column. In PVC, the 11 ml bore size and 9 cm length and a total packing height of 13 mm provides easy handling.
2. Application of uniform pressure, effectively removes the interfering substances without the need for elaborate vacuum assembly required for earlier minicolumns.
3. The solvent system consisting of hexane, chloroform and tetrahydrofuran effectively, removes residual fat and any closed substances that could interfere with the fluorescence of aflatoxin. Hexane has a stabilizing effect on the aflatoxin binding.
4. The binding of aflatoxins on to the florisil layer is enhanced due to increased surface area of the florisil layer.

5. The PMC the advantage of extending the chemical confirmatory tests of aflatoxin on to the minicolumn.

The PMC has been collaboratively tested to evaluate its practical application and extent of variation among analysts of different public health analytical laboratories in India. The results indicated a high degree of reproducibility and repeatability of the method. (6).

The PMC can therefore, be used as a rapid screening and detection method for aflatoxins particularly inpublic health analytical laboratories of the State Government which have to manutorily analyse samples of agricultural commodities suspected to be contaminated with aflatoxins.

REFERENCES

1. Barabalok, R., Colburn, C.R. and Smith, R.J. (1974). Rapid screening method for examining corn and corn-derived products for possible aflatoxin contamination. J. Assoc. Off. Anal. Chem. *57:* 746-766.
2. Holadya, E.C. (1981). Minicolumn chromatography : State of the Art. J. Amer. Oil Chem. Soc. *58:* 931A-934A.
3. Official Methods of Analysis (1984). 14th Ed. AOAC, Arlington, VA, 478-494.
4 Romer, T.R. (1975). Screening methods for the detection of aflatoxins in mixed feeds and other agricultural commodities with subsequent confirmation and quantitative measurement of aflatoxin in positive samples. J. Assoc. Off. Anal. Chem. *58:* 500-506.
5. Romer, T.R. (1984). Chromatographic techniques for mycotoxins. In "Food constituents and food residues: Their chromatographic determination". J.E. Lawrence (Ed.) Mercel Dekker, Inc. N.Y. pp 370.
6. Sashidhar, R.B., Ramakrishna, Y. and Bhat, R.V. (1988). Rapid detection of aflatoxins by pressure minicolumn technique. Anal. Lett. *21*: 507-519.
7. Sashidhar, R.B. and Narsinga Rao, B.S. (1988). Non-Competitive enzyme linked immunosorbent assay for detection of aflatoxin B1. Ind. J. Exp. Biol. 26: 984-989.
8. Sashidhar, R.B., Bhat, R.V and Vasanthi, S. (1989). Rapid detection of aflatoxin by pressure minicolumn technique: A collaborative trial. Curr. Sci. *58*: 882-885
9. WHO-IARC (1982). Environmental carcinogens; Selected methods of analysis, 5-Some Mytoxin. International Agency for research on Cancer, World Health Organization, Geneva, Switzerland.

Indian J. Anim, Sci. **42**(8): 622-24 Angust 1972

CHAPTER

26

FUNGAL HEPATITIS IN POULTRY: A NOTE

Shaik Meera Mohiuddin
College of Veterinary Sciences, Rajendranagar, Hyderabad, Andhra Pradesh

Avian aspergillosis is the commonest fungus responsible for pulmonary lesion in birds, but its occurrence in live is rare, (Raja *et al.*, 1965). Witter and Chute, 1952). In this communication occurrence of hepatic aspergillosis in pullet is reported.

A single White Leghorn pullet belonging to the College Poultry Exam was bought for post-mortem examination. Necrotic lesion was noticed only on the surface of the liver. The lesions from different sites were collected for histopathological examination. For staining procedures, hematoxyling and eosin, Massion's trichrome, Gomori's reticulum, alcian blue periodic acid-Shiff and Grecord modification of Gomori's silver methneamine staining procedures were used.

On gross examination, changes were found only in the liver, which was slightly enlarged and congested. It presented multiple greyish-white casketing nodules of variable size (2 to 6 man diameter). A variable degree of congestion was also found in the remaining organs and tissues. Histologically, the liver presented granulomatus lesions with central necroflammatory exudate, including polymorphonuclear leucocytes, lymphocytes and epithelioid cells. They were surrounded by a well-defined fibroblastic proliferation. The hepatic parenchymas at the periphery of the lesions were compressed. Sinusoids were dilated. There was a variable degree of periportal fibrosis and chronic periophelibits of the branches of portal veins. There was increase in the reticulum fibres, which radiated from the portal tracts into the liver. Multiple fungal hyphae were found amongst the cells of the inflammatory exudate of the granulomatus lesions. They were PAS-positive and alcinophilic. They became more conspicuous in the sections stained with the lesions, in general, conformed to the classical description of mycotic granulomata (Chute, 1965). However, calcification (Ainsworth and Austwick 1959) and giant cell reaction (Nieberle, 1923): Rajan *et al.,* 1965) were not found in any of them.

The identification of the fungus was based on the microscopical appearance of the organisms observed in tissue sections (Fig 1, 2). The fungal hyphae in the lesions are septate and almost sphericla in appearance with dichotmous branching characterisitc of aspergillus in tissues, as reported earlier (Norman, 1968; Soitys, 1963).

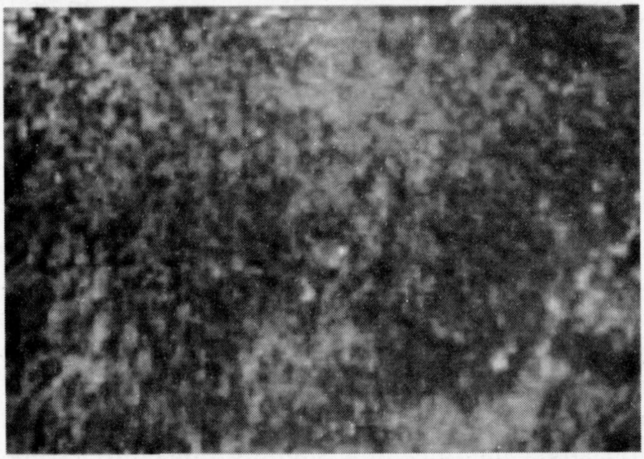

Fig. 1. Caseonecrotic lesion showing fungus surrounded by proliferation of fibroblastic and inflammatiory cells. Hepatic cells are congested and necrotic. H. & E. X 100.

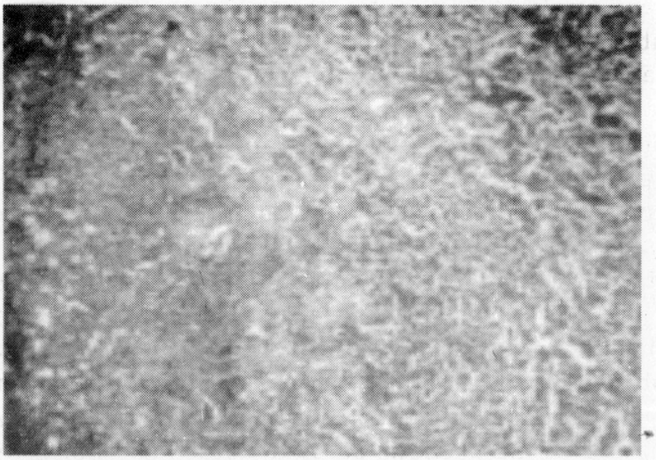

Fig. 2. Fungal hyphae inthe lesion. Silver methane amine stain. X 100.

ACKNOWLEDGEMENTS

The author is thankful to Dr. D. Krishna Murthy, Senior Research Officer (Pathology), National Institute of Nutrition, Hyderabad, for his constant help and guidance.

REFERENCES

Ainsworth, G.C. and Austwick, P.K. C. 1959. *Fungal Disease of Animals* Commonwealth Agricultural Bureaux, Farnham Royal Bucks, England.

Chute, H.L. 1995. *Disease Caused by fungi in Diseases of Poultry.* (Ed.) Biester, H.E. and Schwartre, L.H. 5th edn, pp. 494. The Iowa State University Press, Ames Iowa, U.S.A.

Nieberle, K. 1923. Die lingenasper gillose. In *Toest E. Spoz. Path. Anat. der. Hausticre.R. Choetz. Berlin.* **3** : 804 (*fide* Ainsworth and Austwick, 1959).

Norman F. Cant. 1968. *Miscellaneous Mycoses in Zinsser Microbiology.* (Ed.) David T. Smith, Norman, F. Cant and Hilda Pope Willett, 14th edn, pp. 1180. Appleton, Country Crofts Division of Meredit Corporation, New York.

Rajan, A., Seshadri, S.J., Chandrasekharan Nair, K.P. and Rai, B.N. 1965. Avian aspergillosis: studies on natural cases and experimental transmission. *Indian vet. J.* 42 : 390.

Soitys, B. 1963. *Bacteria and Fungi Pathogenic to Man and Animals.* 1st edn, pp. 475. Bailliere, Tindal & Cox, London.

Witter, J.F. and Chute, H.L. 1952. *Aspergillosis* in turkeys. *J. Am. med. Ass.* **122:** 387. In *Diseases of Poultry* (Ed.) Biester, H.E. and Schwarte, L.H. 5thed, pp. 496. The Iowa State University Press, Ames, Iowa, U.S.A.

CHAPTER 27

MOULDS AND MYCOTOXINS IN POULTRY DISEASES

Dr. Shaik Meera Mohiuddin,
M.V.Sc. (Path), Ph.D. Jr. Poultry Pathologist, A.I.C.R.P. On Poultry for Eggs, Rajendranagar, Hyderabad.

Disease caused by moulds and mycotoxins in farm animals have been realised long back, however it is neglected a possible aetiological agent in diseases of farm animals with an exception to Ergotism. A variety of names such as moulds corn disease, blind staggers, yellow liver disease, dumb disease have been referred in mycotoxicosis (Wilson *et al* (1967).

Mouldy contamination of cereals, groundnuts and other feed stuffs has been frequently reported (Forgags, 1965., Scott., 1965., Nelson *et al.*, 1968). Feeding of such contaminated feed stuffs lead to the problems several kinds of toxicosis.

"Yellow rice" toxicity in Japan has been traced to contamination with fungi *Pencilleum islandicum* (Urageuchi *et al.*, 1061). Fungal toxins of *pithmyces Chartarum* was responsible for facial eczema in sheep of New Zealand (Lancaster, 1969). Pencillium spp. was experimentally shown to be associated with nervous disorders (Miyake *et al.*, 1940). In Russia outbreaks of mycotoxicosis causing alimentary toxic alenkia (ATA) was recorded during World War II (Joffe, 1965). Extensive haemorrhagic lesions in calves fed with contaminated feed, with *Aspergillus fumigatus* was described by Caroll *et al.*, (1955). Burnside *et al.*, (1957) described the clinical and pathological features in several epizootics of mycotoxicosis in swine, horses and goats. *Pencillium rubrum* causing heptatotoxic haemorrhagic was noticed in several laboratory animals and in dogs (Wilson and Wilson, 1962). Haemorrhagic syndrome in chicks, ducklings and turkey poults were caused by *Aspergillus* and *Pencillium* spp. (Forgags and Caroll, 1955., Mircocha *et al,* 1968). frequently deaths in Turkey poults and chicks has been reported due to the feeding of contaminated feed with *pencilium* and *Fusarium* spp. (Firgaes *et al.* 1962., Meronuck *et al.*, 1970). Recently 493 deaths in 1000 laying hens were by feeding moudly corn within 48 hours, and a reduction of 5% eggs production in survivers, in America (Hamilton 1972).

Mouldiness results in unpleasant flavour and undesirable changes in the food products. Certain molds have the capacity to synthesise certain chemical substances which will be poisonous to the animals when consumed. Even more important when things of mycotixin, is that it exits in the feed even after the destrul of moulds, thus creating a difficulty in identifying moulds corn and further mycotoxins are relatively to all types of treatments. Another important feature of mycotoxicosis is that it does not gives an idea of the size of economic loss, caused, but such dramatic cutostraphic cases will occur infrequently. Apart from their direct hazards to the health of animals, the toxic substances at times will be excreted through meat, milk and eggs and cause a serious problem in humans.

Since the outbreak of Turkey "x" disease in Britain during the year 1960, a worldwide attention has been attached for a thorugh investigation of mycotoxicosis. This has led to the discovery and detailed investigation of aflatoxicosis in groundnuts and other feeds contaminated by *Aspergillus falvus* and *Parasitieus.* A group of metabolic products produced by these fungi were termed as aflatoxins.

Fungi growth

Aspergillus belonging to the family Aspergillae. These are the major cause of damage, spoilage of stored grains. The damage done by the stored fungi depends upon the storage conditions. It grows rapidly in relatively greater moisture than most other moulds and requires a temperature of 28-35°C and relative humidity of 80-85%. Such favourable conditions are mostly present in ground kernels and defeated meal with moisture content from 0-10%. The spoilage of storage grains then depends upon the (1) storage conditions (2) The extent to which grains already is invaded by storage fungi (3) length of time of grains to be stored (Christensen, 1957).

Aflatoxin producing fungal strains are widely dispersed in air and soil and are capable of growth apart from groundnuts. It has been reported from rice corn, soyabeans, oats, wheat and mutton.

Several groups of investigators (Sargeant *et al.*, 1961., Nesbitt *et al.*, 1962., Vanderzitden *et al.* 1962) have reported reagarding the isolation and characterisation of four closely related compounds with toxic properties. The molecular formulae established from elementary analysis and spectometric determination are (Hartley *et al,*1963).

$B_1 = C_{17} H_{12}$ 06, G_1=$C_{17} H_{12}$ 07

$B_2 = C_{17} H_{14}$ 06 G_2=$C_{17} H_{12}$ 07

Aflatoxins are strongly fluorescent in ultraviolet light. Aflatoxin B_1 and B_2 are so named because they emit visible blue light under ultraviolet light while G_1 and G_2 flouresence green.

Metabolism:

Knowledge about the metabolic fate of aflatoxins might help in assessing the extent to which edible animal tissue to their products may become contaminated with the toxins or their derivatives when animals were fed rations, containing the compounds. It may also help in understanding the biochemical mechanisms underlying their biological effects, species differences in responsiveness and tissue specificity of the toxins.

Metabolism of aflatoxin was studied in detailed animals *viz* rats (Butler and Clifford, 1965., Flank *et al.,* 1965., Shaik and Wogan 1965., Patterson and Allcroft, 1970), Sheep (Allcroft *et al* 1966., Nabney *et al.,* 1977., Petterson *et al.,* 1968) and guinea pig (Patterson and Allcroft, 1970).

Following the administration of the toxin orally or intraperitoneally it was absorbed into blood and could be demonstrated in liver within 30 minutes and in about 60 level it reached its maximum level in their liver (Butler and Clifford, 1965). Earliest ultrastructural alterations were found in liver cells lying in the vicinity of red blood cells, hence it was transported by the red cells (Theron, 1965-Theron *et al.*1965). The toxin was absorbed into circulation from intestinal mucosa in an unaltered form and the metabolic alterations will occur in liver alone (Butler and Clifford, 1965).

Cows fed the toxic meal excreted in their milk a factor that was toxic to duckling, which was present in rennet precipitated casein fractions. They are M1 and M2, hydroxylated derivatives of aflatoxin B_1 and B_2.

Only 4.52% of the administered dosage, was extracted through urine 1.55/5, feaces 2.79 and 0.18% in milk, 85% of total extraction occurred within 48 hours in milk and urine and no toxin was found in 6 hours respectively. (Allcroft and Robert 1968).

Aflatoxin tend to undergo two types of metabolic conversions: (1) Ring hydroxylation given rise to monohydroxylated derivative (aflatoxin M.), seen in milk, excepted and liver (2) O-demethylation, a major degradation pathway giving rise to phenolic derivative, whose subsequent metabolic fate was unknown. These processes occurs in the liver of the treated animals suggesting the relative retention of the compound in that organ and also localisation of biochemical and histological effects in liver (Wogan, 1965).

The differences in susceptibility of different species was attributed to the (1) presence of enzymes inhibitors (Axelord, 1956), (2) Unstable enzyme systems (Cochine and Axelrod, 1959) and (3) Variation in cell permeability (Portam *et al.* 1970) to the toxin.

Biochemical effects:

It was reported that aflatoxins acts primarlyon metabolic systems located in mitochondria and particularly on dehydrogenases like (i) succinic dehydrogenase (ii) Glycerophosphate dehydrogenase (iii) electranfer chains and oxidative phosphorilation mechanisms (Abrams, 1965), while Tulpule (1966) showed that microson enzymes of the liver cells were affected earlier than mitochondrial enzymes.

A decrease in the incorporation of C_{14} labelled leucine into protein of the liver slice of rat and ducklings led aflatoxin B_1, suggested a suppression of the synthesis of protein by the toxin (Smith, 1963). Following aflatoxin B_2, feeding hydrocartizone failed to induce hepatic tryptophan pyrolase or protein synthesis, suggesting suppression of enzyme synthesis by the toxin (Wogan and Friedman, 1965). Suppression of nuclear RNA synthesis and cortizone induced tryptophan pyrolase in the over of rat poisoned with aflatoxin B1 suggest an inhibition of the synthesis of messenger RNA by the toxin (Clifford and Ress 1966., Friedman and Wogan 1966). As such the sequence of events following the administration of the toxin were; The toxin after entering liver cells gets concentrated in the nucleus, binds with DNA and inhibit the RNA polymerase. The reduction in RNA synthesis is resumably due to suppression of messenger RNA synthesis as suggested by the inhibition of tryptophan pyrolase. The inhibition of messenger RNA could be effected in reduced synthesis of protein about 15 minutes later (Clifford and Rees, 1966).

In various species studied, liver protein decreased, lipid increases and hepatic liver glycogen came down. A decrease in hepatic glocogen could be due to a decrease in the ectivitities of oxidative phosphorilase and glucose-6-phosphatose, which is a part of overall suppression of protein synthesis by the toxin (Tulpure *et al.* 1965, Madhavan *et al.*, 1965, Carnaghan, 1966, Shank and Wogan, 1966, Madhavan and Rao, 1967, Gumbhann and Williams, 1969., Allcroft and Lewis 1963, Carnaghan *et al.* 1966).

Accumalation of fat in liver cells were explained on the basis of failure of its transport mechanism rather than its increased synthesis, for lypoproteins are known to transport the lipids from the liver cells, whose synthesis is affected (Lombordi, 1966., John and Miller, 1969., Wogan and Raymond, 1970). The haemorrhagic phenomena often encountered in aflatoxicosis may be attributable to the impairment of the activities of Coagulation factors VII and X and IX (Upcott, 1970) and increased capillary permeability due to loss of tissue strength as a result of degradation of preformed, structural elements by the release of lysosomal enzymes like acid phosphatase (Tangtung *et al.*, 1970).

Histological Changes

Since the initial discovery and isolation, aflatoxins has been evaluated in wide variety of biological system than any other mycotoxins. Aflatoxins are potent hepatotoxins. The toxins were reported to be Teratogenic, Mutagenic, and Carcinogenic (Legator, 1969) and antimytotic in activity (Green, 1968).

The effects of aflatoxin may be acute or chronic depending primarly on the dosage and frequency of exposure. Secondarly it depends on status of the individuals. Young ones in general were more susceptible than older (Tulpule *et al.* 1964, Allcroft 1965, Cuthbertsen *et al.*, 1967, Legator 1969., O'gara and Kelly, 1967) Males are more susceptible than females (Butler, 1964b, Wogan, 1965., Wogan and Newberne, 1967., Newberne and Williams, 1969). Pregnancy (Allcroft, 1964, Butler and Wigglesworth, 1966, Butler and Wigglesworth, 1966) and low protein diet (Madhavan *et al.*, 1965. Madhavan and Gopalan, 1965) enhances the susceptibility. The toxicity influences (Madhavan, 1967). The species, for ducklings were suceptible than chicks and among form animals sheep is resistant to cattle. Among the Avian species the highly suscepitible ones in their sequential order wee ducklings, turkey poults and chickens. Reduced weight grain with 2% mortality was reported in broiler chickens with 15% toxic meal for a period of twelve weeks (Allcroft, 1965) Aflatoxin at a level of 2.5, 5.0 and 10 ppm in the diet decreases growth rate an enlargement of liver spleen and pancreas (Smith and Hamiltin, 1970). Hepatic tumor develop in ducklings fed a diet containing 5% toxic meal over a period of 14 months (Carnaghan, 1963).

In majority of the species of animals tested death usually occurred within a few days following administration of toxin. The first sign of the disease in bird is in appetence and poor growth rate. Duckling may start eating but subsequent lose their interest in food. Crop usually empty. A cry of discomfort will be noticed. A consicuous feature seen in White coloration of the legs and feet, and ducklings showing these lesion were often severally lame. Finally they develop atoxia followed by convulsions and diet in opishatonus.

Gross lesions depends upon the severity of the toxicity and survival time. In birds dying within week the liver is putty coloured, slightly enlarged. Kidneys were pale, slightly swollen with few diffusely scattered haemorrhages and frequent patachial haemorrhages on pancreas. In those survived more than three weeks, the liver was ample reticulated throughout its substance leading to shrngkage to cirrhosis, associated with ascitis. In still advance cases subcutaneous haemorrhages in unfeathered parts of the leg and web causing published dicoloration in white skinned birds. At times a glelutinous subcutaneous exudate may be noticed.

The histological change may be acute or chronic. In acute cases there is diffuse degenerative changes of the hepatic parenclyma. The cells swells and became vacuolated. The nuclei are enlarged and showed karyorexis and Karyolysis and finally leading to liver fell necrossi with mononeuclear cell in filtration. In chronic cases there is variable degree of fatty change of liver cells, bile ductular and mesenclymal proliferation leading to biliary fibrosis and finally cirrhosis with the formation of pseudolobules and regenerating nodules.

The hepatic changes in various species of animals were more or less similar in nature. They, however, varied in their distribution in different species. Liver changes in ducklings, turkeys, monkeys, and chickens were periportal while in guinea pig, dog and Bove. were centrilobular. The knowledge of mycotoxins and their importance to forming and allied industry will help in preventing their contamination. An increased awareness of mycotoxins and their implictions to animals and human health will benefit us all.

REFERENCES

Arrams, L., (1065) : J.S. Afri. Vet. Med. Ass. *36*: 5.

Allcroft, R., and Lewis, G. (1963): Vet Rec. *75*: 487.

Allcroft, R., (1964): "Mycotoxins in Foodstuffs" Proceedings of the symposium held at Massachusette institute of Technology March 18 and 19th.

Allcroft, R. (1965): Mycotoxins in Food stuffs (Wogan Edt.) M.I.T. Press, Cambridge, Massachusette.

Axelord, J. (1956): Bichen, J. 634.

Burniside, J.E., Sippel, W.L., Forgags, J., Carroll, W.T., Atwoot, M.B., and Doll, E.R. (1957): Amer. J. Vet.Res *18* : 817.

Butler, W.H. (1964b): Brit. J. Cancer, *18*: 756.

Butler, W.H. and Caroll, W.T. Forgags, J., Herring, A.S. and Mahludt. B.G., (1955), Vet. Med. *50* : 210.

Cambell, T.C. (1970), Biophys, Acta, *208*: 487.

Clifford, J.I. (1965), Nature *206* : 1045.

Butler, W.H. and Wigglesworth, J.S. (1966) : Brit. J. of Expt. Pathol. XLVII : 242.

Carnaghan, R.B.A., Hartley, R.D., and O'Kelly, J. (1963) Nature *200* : 1101.

Carnaghan, R.B.A., Lewis, G., Patterson, D.S.P. and Allcroft, R. (1966), Path. Vet 3 : 601.

Christensen, C.M. (1957) : Botan-Rev. *23* : 108.

Clifford, J.I. and Rees, K.R. (1966) Nature, *209* : 312.

Cochin, J. and Axelord, J. (1959), J. Phramae *125*: 105

Cuthbertson, W.F. J., Laursen, A.C., and Pratt. D.A.H. (1969), Brit. J. Natr. *21*: 893.

Falk, H.L., Thompson, S.J., Kotin, P. (1965). Proc. Amer. Cancer Res. *6* : 18.

Forgags, J., and Carroll, W.T. (1955), Vet. Med. *50* : 172.

Forgags, J., Koch, K., Carroll,W.T.A White Stevens, R. H. (1962), Avian. Dis. *6* : 363.

Green, S. (1068), Nature, *220* : 931.

Gumbhann, M.R. and Williams, S.N. (1969), Toxicity Appl. Pharmacol. *15* : 393.

Hamilton, Pat. B. (1972), Master Manual or Molds and Mycotoxins, *P* 3.

Hartley, R.D., Nestitt, B.F., and O'Kelly, J (1963), Nature *198* : 1056.

Joffe, A.Z. (1965), "Mycotoxins in food stuffs" (Wo. Edt)., *P*. 77. M.I.T Press Cambridge, Massachusette.

John, D.W. and Miller, L.L. (1969), Biochem. Pharmacol. *18* : 1135.

Lombordi, B., (1966) Lab. Invest. *15* : 11.

Lancaster, M.C. (1969), Proc. Nutr. Soc. 28 : 203.

Lancaster, M.C. (1969), Aflatoxin (Goldblatt. ed.) P. 107 Acad, Press. New York London.

Madhavan, T.V. Rao, S.K. and Tulpule, P. (1983), Ind. J.Med. Res. *53* : 984.

Madhavan, T.V. and Gopalan C. (1965), Arch, Path, *79* : 466.

Madhavan, T.V. (1967), J. Path. and Bact. 93 : 443.

Meronuck, R.A., Garren, K.H., Christensen, C.M. Nelson, C.H. and Fern Bates (1970), Amer, J, Vet Res. *31* : 551.

Mirocha, C.J., Christensen, C.M. and Nelson G.M. (1968), biotechnol- Bioeng. *10* : 469.

Miyake, I., Naito, H., and Tsunoda, H. (1940, Beikoko Riyo, Keukyuto. Hokou., *1* : 1.

Nabney, J., Burbage, M.B., Allcroft, R., and Lewis G. (1967), Fd. Cosmet, Toxicol. *5* : 11.

Nelson, G.H., Christensen, C.M. and Microcha, (1969),Toxocol and appl. Pharmacol. *12* : 325.

Nesbitt, B.F. O'Kelly , J. Sargeant, K. and Sheridan, A. (1962), Nature *195* : 1062.

Nesbitti, B. F. and O'Kelly, J. (1963).

New Berne, P.M. and Williams, G (1969), Arch. Environ, Health *19* , 489.

O'gara, R.W. and Kelly, M.G. (1969), Tropic and Gogr. Med. *21* ; 1.

Pattersen, D.S.P. and Allcroft, R. (1970) Food Cosmet. Toxicol. *8* : 43.

Portman, R.S. Plowman, K.M. and Rees, K.R. (1966). Proc. Roy. Soc. Med., *9*: 755.

Segeant, K., Allcroft R., and Carnaghan, R.B.A. (1961), Vet. Rec., *73* : 865.

Scott, D.B. (1965), Mycopath : Mycol. Appl. *25* : 213.

Shank, R.G and Wogan, G.N. (1985), Fed. Proc. *24* : 627.

Shank, R.G. and Wogan, G.N. (1966), Toxicol. Appl. Pharmacol. *9*: 468.

Smith, R.H. (1963), Biochem, J., *88*: 50.

Tasgtung, Hs., Donaldson, W.E. and Hamilton, P.B. (1970), Biochem. Biophys. Acta, 222 : 665.

Theron, J.J. (1965), Lab. Invest. *14* : 1586.

Theron, J.J., Lie Bernberg, N. and Joubert. H.J.B., (1965), Nature, *206* : 908.

Tulpule, P.G., Madhavan, T.V. (1964). Lancet, *1* : 962, Tulpule, P.G. (1965).

Tulpule, (1066), Annual Report of N.I.N. Hyd.

Upcott. D.H. (1970), Ebl. Vet. Med. Asso. *17* : 278.

Uraguchi, K,, Tatsuno.T., Sakai, F., Tsukioka, M., Sakai, Y., Yonemits, U.O., ITO, H., Mixake, M., Saito, M., Enomoto, N., Saikata, T., and Isaiko, T. (1961), Japan J. Exp., Md. *31*: 1.

Vanderzitden, A.G.M. Blanch Koelen Mid, W.A.A. Bioldinga., J., Barrett, C.B. Ord. W.O. and Philip, J. (1962), Nature, *195* : 1060.

Wilson, B.J. and Wilson, C.H. (1962), J.Bact. , *84* : 283.

Wilson, *et al.* 1967.

Wogan, G.N., (1965) "Mycotoxins in food stuffs" (Wogan ed.) P. 163, M.I.T. Press. Cambridge, Massachusette.

Wogan, G.N., and Fridman, M.A. (1965) Fed. Proc. *24* : 627.

Wogan, G.N. and New Berne, P.M. (1967), Cancer, es. *27*: 2370.

Wogan, G.N. and Ramond, S.P. (1970). Annals of New York Acad. Sci. *174* : 623.

Woodham, A.A. and Dawson, R. 1966. The effect of heat on defatted groundnut flour. *Proc. Nutr. Soc.* **25:** 8.

Zombade, S.S. 1977. *Studies on the relationship between biological and laboratory methods of protein quality evaluation.* Ph. D. Thesis, Punjab Agricultural University, Ludhiana.

Zambade, S.S. and SATHE, B. S. 1979. Variation in nutrient content and protein quality of fish-meal and groundnut-cake, *Indian J. Amin. Sci.* **49** : 98-103.

Zombade, S.S., Lodhi, G.N. and Ichhponani, J.S. 1980a. Evaluation of Protein quality of poultry feeding stuffs, I. Comparison of Chick biossays, *J. agric, Sci., Comb.* **94** : 105-10.

Zombade, S.S. Doghi, G.N. and Ichhponani, J.S. 1980b. Evaluation of protein quality of poultry feeeding stuffs, 2-Fish and meal. *J. agric, Sci. Camb.* **94** : 111-16.

Zombade, S.S. Lodhi, G.N. and Ichhponani, J.S. 1980c. Evaluation of protein quality of poultry feeding stuffs, 3. Oilseed cakes. *J. agric, Sci. Camb.* **94** 117-20.

CHAPTER 28

STUDIES ON THE EFFECTS OF AFLATOXIN ON ANTIBODY SYNTHESIS AGAINST RANKIKHET DISEASE VACCINE IN CHICKS

Shaik Meera Mohiuddin, D. Mahendranath, B. Yadgiri and S.R. Ahmed

College of Veterinary Science Andhra Pradesh Agricultural University, Hyderabad, Andhra Pradesh 500 003.

ABSTRACT

Feeding of aflatoxin @ 100 mg daily/chick for 14 days prior to vaccination for Ranikhet disease (RI) and a further feeding of 21 days after RD vaccination did not affect the haemotological parameters studied. The effect of feeding 100 and 200 mg of aflatoxin daidy for 14 days before RD vaccination was similar, but further feeding of aflatoxin @ 200 mg for 21 days after RD vaccine resulted in increased serum-alkaline-phosphatase activity, increased RBC's fragility marked testicular attroph and decrease in antibody without any change in other parameters studied. Administration of vitamin A gave protection against aflatoxin, but failed to enhance the immunity. Thus feeding of aflatoxin at a level of 0.1 ppm to poultry during the stress of vaccination did not interfere with any biochemical activity, whereas feeding with 0.2 ppm interfered with biochemical activities.

Little work has been done in India on the effects of aflatoxin against antibody formation, especially against tviral diseases. Also not much information is available regarding the feeding of excessive amount of vitamin A on the development of immunity againt Ranikhet diseases. Grains unfit for human consumption are used in the ration of livestock and poultry. Sufficient information is also lacking regarding the permissible levels of the contaminated grains that can be utilized in rations of poultry without any untoward effects. In this communication, an experimental model is planned to study these aspects.

MATERIALS AND METHODS

Seventy-five day-old male chicks were reared for 4-weeks.

Random samples of blood were collected for haematology. Faecal samples are examined for any parasitic and protoxoal infection. The chicks were weighed and divided into 5 chicks were weighed and divided into 5 groups of 15 chicks in each group. The number of chicks in each group and the schedule of treatment are shown in Table 1.

Table 1. Experimental model

Group	Treatment
1	Propylenedglycol 1ml/bird/day
2.	100 mg of aflatoxin in 1 ml propyleneglycol/bird/day
3.	200 mg of aflatoxin in 1 ml propyleneglycol/bird/day
4.	100 mg of aflatoxin in 1 ml of propyleneglycol + vit. A 1,000 IU/bird/day
5.	200 mg of aflatoxin in 1 ml of propyleneglycol + vit. A. 1,000 IU/bird/day

All these chicks were fed with ration purchased from a local feed manufacturer. Cyrstalline preparation of aflatoxin was dissolved in propyleneglycol so as to give a concentration of 100 and 200 mg per ml. Vitamin of 100 and 200 mg per ml. Vitamin A solution was prepared in water so as to give 1,000 IU per ml. Every morning the birds were fed as per schedule for 14 days. The feed samples were subjected to ethenol extraction and analysed by thin-layer chromatographic method to detect any feed contamination with aflatoxin.

On the 15th day birds were weighed. Blood samples were collected for analysis of packed-cell volume (PCV), haemoglobin (Hb), total red blood cells (RBC), white blood cell (WBC), count, thrombocytic and differential counts. Blood was also collected from random samples of 10 chicks in all the 5 groups to determine prevaccinated serum antibody titres. Then all chicks were vaccinated Ranikhet disease (R_2B strain) vaccine. After vaccination on the 15th day, 9 birds of the groups 2 to 5 were continued with their respective treatments for another 21 days and the remaining chicks were maintained on grower ration alone. On the seventh day of first vaccination to boost up the production of antibodies, another dose of

RD ('R_2B' strain) vaccination was given to all the chicks. After 14 days of second vaccination all the chicks were weighed and sacrificed. Blood was collected for haematological analysis and estimation for serum antibody titres by haemagglutination-inhibition test (HAI). Serum-alkaline phophatase (Bodansky, 1932), erythrocyte sedimentation rate and fragity test (oxmotic fragility method) were also determined in the birds which received toxin till sacrificed. Detailed post-mortem examination was bursa Fabricius were collected for detailed histopathology. The haematological findings, serum-alkaline phosphatase, antibody titres and weights of the testes in all the groups were analysed using analysis of variance technique and 'T' test.

RESULTS AND DISCUSSION

There was no significant difference in body weights recorded in the fourth week,14 days after toxin feeding and at killing between the groups (Table 2). Feeding off 100 and 200 mg of toxin daily with or without added dose of vitamin A for 14 days only did not present any significant differences in PCV, Hb, RBC, WBC, thrombocytes and

Table 2. Body weights (g) of birds 35 days after feeding aflatoxin

Group	Initial	14 days after toxin feeding	killing 14 days after feeding toxin	killing 35 days after feeding toxin
1	572.1±4.93 (15)	797.92®4.91 (15)	1161.7±15.54 (6)	1177.5±1027 (9)
2	522.07±4.19 (15)	770.0±7.12 (15)	1093.1±12.43 (6)	7784.4±7.11 (9)
3	542.71±8.21 (15)	746.57±7.97 (15)	1025±11.57 (6)	1196.4±17.75 (9)
4.	545.07±5.89 (15)	723.4±6.68 (15)	1062±9.34 (6)	1165.0±11.48 (9)
5	579.5±4.94 (15)	770.92±6.71 (15)	1003.7±19.30 (6)	1210.0±20.20 (9)

Mean ± S.E.

Number of parentheses indicates sample size

differential counts, and at the time of killing between the groups 1 to 5. Similarly these was no significant difference in these values between groups 1 and 5, which were continued with toxin after 14 days till the time of killing (Table 3). Chicks receiving aflatoxin with or without added dose of vitamin A did not difference in their haematological values on killing between groups 1 to 5 (Table 3). A comparison was made between the groups receiving aflatoxn with and without added vitamin A before vaccination and continued after vaccination. No significant difference was observed in these values (group 2 to 3) (Table 4). Erythrocyte sedimentation rate in groups 1 to 5 which were on treatment on continued feeding, did not show any significant difference, while the fragile test showed significance.

EFFECT OF AFLATOXIN ON RD VACCINE

Differences ($P<0.01$). Group 1 was significantly different from groups 2 to 5 but there were no differences between G_2, G_3 and G_5, and G_3 G_4 and G_5 (Table 5). Antibody titres were significantly different between the 5 groups ($P<0.01$). No significant differences were found between groups 1 and 3, but they were different from groups 1 to 3, but they were different from groups 4 to 5 (Table 5). Serum-alkaline-phosphatase activity did not show any difference between groups 1, 2, 4 and 5, but group 3 was significantly ($P<0.01$) different from the remaining groups (Table 5). On autopsy significant ($P<0.01$) reduction in testicular weights in groups 3 and 5 was noticed, but there were no weight differences in groups, 1, 2 and 4 (Table 5). All the livers from the groups did not present any significant histological changes.

The effect of the toxin depends upon the dosage, protein status in the diet and the species. Young animals are more susceptible than adults. A diet poor in protein increases the susceptibility of the animals. Aflatoxin interferes with the sythesis of proteins (Smith, 1963), brings about a qualitative change in serum protein (Annan*et al.*, 1964; Brown and Abrahams, 1965), arrests the mitosis in tissue cultures of leucocytes (Dolimpo *et al.*, 1968) and affects the hepatic cell division in cirrhosis (Loweustein and Lee, 1966). From the foregoing information, it is reasonable to pressume that alatoxin any interfere with the production of immunity. This problem has much economical and practical significance in the developing poultry industry, since usually very young birds are vaccinated and the poultry rations are frequently contaminated with moulds.

Continuous feeding of aflatoxin at 100 mg for 21 days after RD

Table 3. Haemotological values in chicks

Groups		PCV (%)	Hb (g %)	RBCs (million/mm^2)	Thromboytes (Thousands/mm^3)	WBCs (Thousands/ mm^3)	Neutrophills (%)	Lymphocytes (%)	Monocytes (%)
1.	(a)	44.1±0.89	12.2±0.06	4.40±1.12	18.8±0.43	20.1±0.66	18±0.31	2±0.01	
		(8)	(8)	(8)	(8)	(8)	(8)	(8)	(7)
	(b) and	35.7±0.24	12.1±0.21	5.53±0.17	18.2±0.35	24±0.56	72±0.76	6±0.47	
	(c)	(12)	(11)	(12)	(11)	(12)	(12)	(12)	(9)
2.	(a)	41.1±0.49	11.40±0.52	5.11±0.11	28.0±0.98	27.3±0.76	11±1.19	88±1.23	1±0.08
		(6)	(6)	(6)	(6)	(6)	(6)	(6)	(6)
	(b)	38.50±0.24	10.9±0.07	5.14±0.07	18.3±0.34	20.7±0.11	32±0.94	64±0.73	5±0.63
		(6)	(6)	(6)	(6)	(6)	(6)	(6)	(6)
	(c)	39.01±0.68	10.9±0.18	5.07±0.21	18.4±0.40	19.6±0.17	27±1.32	79±1.11	6±1.16
		(6)	(6)	(6)	(6)	(6)	(6)	(6)	(6)
3.	(a)	44.9±0.67	10.1±0.09	4.02±0.07	21.8±0.73	21.1±1.46	22±0.88	72±0.67	7±0.42
		(5)	(6)	(6)	(5)	(5)	(6)	(6)	(6)
	(b)	38.01±0.40	10.6±0.07	5.8±0.08	15.6±0.24	16.4±0.46	30±0.25	69±0.20	2±
		(6)	(6)	(6)	(6)	(6)	(6)	(6)	(3)
	(c)	39.8±0.42	12.4±0.45	5.29±0.10	17.6±0.44	18.4±0.36	28±0.31	71±0.31	2±0.16
		(6)	(6)	(6)	(6)	(6)	(6)	(6)	(3)
4.	(a)	43.6±0.63	11.3±0.33	11.29±0.11	17.4±0.45	19.71±0.62	13±0.59	86±0.70	2±0.2
		(6)	(5)	(6)	(6)	(5)	(6)	(6)	(4)
	(b)	35.7±0.11	10.6±0.24	5.41±0.18	19.6±0.61	17.7±0.61	29±0.29	70±0.32	3±0.20
		(7)	(7)	(7)	(7)	(7)	(7)	(7)	(2)
	(c)	36.1ê.62	10.7±0.28	4.33±0.14	18.1±0.14	18.6±0.78	24±0.55	75±0.72	3±0.75
		(6)	(6)	(6)	(6)	(6)	(6)	(6)	(2)
5.	(a)	42.6±0.52	12.4±0.25	4.82±0.66	21.9±0.66	21.9±0.83	32±1.05	64±0.79	5±0.41
	(6)	(5)	(6)	(6)	(6)	(6)	(6)	(3)	
	(b)	39.8±0.81	10.5±0.18	5.85±0.17	17.0±0.52	22.6±0.60	27±0.39	72±0.40	2±
		(6)	(6)	(6)	(6)	(6)	(6)	(6)	(2)
	(c)	39.8±0.26	12.6±0.19	4.68±0.13	19.6±0.63	17.7±0.65	25±0.53	74±0.61	2±0.16
		(6)	(6)	(6)	(6)	(6)	(6)	(6)	(3)

Mean ± S.E.

Number in parentheses indicates sample size

a. In chicks fed toxin for 14 days before vaccination

b. In chicks fed toxin for 14 days vaccination and subsequently maintained on stock diet till sacrifice.

c. In chicks which were on continuous feeding of toxin before and after vaccination till sacrifice.

Table 4. Comparison of haematological values in chicks fed toxin before vaccination and after vaccination at the time of killing.

Group	No. of days toxin was fed	PCV (%)	Hb (g%)	RBCs (thousands/mm^3)	Thrombocyte (thousands /mm^3)	WBCs (thousands / mm^3)	Nuetrophils (%)	Lymphocytes (%)	Monocytes (%)
2.	14 days	37.5±0.58 (6)	10.9±1.83 (6)	5.14±0.17 (6)	18.30±0.83 (6)	20.40±0.5 (6)	32.7±1.39 (6)	64.2±1.79 (6)	4.6±1.40 (5)
	35 days	39.0±1.67 (6)	10.75±0.44 (6)	5.07±0.51 (6)	18.36±0.97 (6)	19.57±0.43 (6)	26.7±.3.24 (6)	69.2±2.72 (6)	6.3±1.55 (6)
3.	14 days	38.0±0.89 (5)	10.6±0.17 (5)	5.80±0.36 (5)	15.6±0.54 (5)	16.4±1.02 (5)	30.0±0.56 (5)	68.8±0.44 (5)	2.0±0 (3)
	35 days	36.6±1.04 (6)	12.4±1.11 (6)	5.29±0.24 (6)	17.6±1.08 (6)	18.4±0.88 (6)	27.8±0.76 (6)	71.3±0.77 (6)	1.7±0.27 (3)
4.	14 days	36.6±0.28 (7)	10.6±0.63 (7)	5.410.46 (7)	19.6±1.60 (7)	17.8±1.66 (7)	29.4±0.78 (7)	69.7±0.85 (7)	3±0.71 (2)
	35 days	36.0±1.52 (6)	10.7±0.69 (6)	4.33±0.33 (6)	18.0±1.00 (6)	15.3±4.74 (6)	24.0±1.35 (6)	75.2±1.77 (6)	20±1.06 (5)
5.	14 days	39.8±1.98 (6)	10.5±0.44 (6)	5.9±0.59 (6)	17.0±1.28 (6)	22.6ë.28 (6)	22.6±1.48 (6)	72.2±1.21 (6)	2±0 (2)
6.	35 days	38.8±0.83 (6)	12.6±0.32 (6)	19.6±1.17 (6)	17.7±1.61 (6)	25.3±1.19 (6)	73.9ë.50 (6)	1.7±0.27 (6)	(3)

Mean ± S.E.
Number in parentheses indicates sample size.

vaccination did not affect the weight gain, erythrocyte sedimentation rate, PCV, Hb, RCB count, thrombocytic count, WBC count, differential count, fragility of RBCs, serum-alkaline phosphatase, antibodies formation and histological changes in chicks, But feeding of 200 mg aflatoxin resulted in increase in serum-alkaline resulted in serum-alkaline-phosphatase activity; however there were no changes in other parameters studies. The tests were markedly atrophied in chicks fed with 200 mg of aflatoxin. Administration of added doses of vitamin A gave protection again the effects of 200 mg of aflatoxin with the result there was no increase in serum-alkaline phosphatase in groups 5. Administration of additional doses of vitamin A during immunization period was reported to increase the immunological response in mice (Jurin and Taunock, 1972). This effect was not noticed in this study.

Table 5. Erythrocyte sedimentation rate, fragility test, antibody test, antibody titres, weight of testis and serum-alkaline phosphatase in chicks kept on toxin before and after vaccination.

Groups	ESR in mm/60 min	Fragility (%)	Antibody titres (HAI units)	Weight of right testis (g)	Serum-alkaline phosphatase (mg/P/100ml/hr)
1	0.87±0.06	0.72±0.008	2958±34	5.30±0.32	904±23.76
	(8)	(9)	(9)	(7)	(6)
2.	1.37±0.05	0.57±0.005	2710±52	5.21±0.37	1043.7±17.76
	(8)	(9)	(9)	(7)	(6)
3.	1.12±0.07	0.62±0.006	2730±32	2.88±0.42	1240.5±14.83
	(8)	(9)	(9)	(7)	(6)
4.	0.93±0.08	0.65±0.006	2399±43	0.11±0.31**	1007.6±17.96
5.	1.37±0.08	0.63±0.007**	2048±29**	0.35±0.04**	1090.5±9.63
	(8)	(9)	(9)	(7)	(6)

Mean ± S.D.
Number in parentheses indicates sample size.
**, P<0.01

ACKNOWLEDGMENTS

We thank Dr. C.V. Reddy, Dean, Faculty of Veterinary Science, for his guidance in carrying out this work.

REFERENCES

Annan, E. Corner, A.H., Magwood, S.K. and Jericho, K. 1964. Electrophoretic and chemical studies n sera of salines following the feeding of toxin groundnut-meal. *Can. J. comp. Med. Vet. Sci.* 28: 264-69.

Bodansky, A. 1932. Phosphatase studies, 1. Determination of inorganic hosphate. beeri low and interfering substances in the Kuttner-Lichtenstein method. *J. biol. Chem.* **99** 197.

Brown, J.M.M. and Abrahams, R. 1965. Biochemical studies on aflatoxicosis. *Ondersteport J. Vet. Res.* **32** : 199.

Dolipio, D., Jacobson, C and Legator, M. 1968. Effects of aflatoxin on human leucocytes. *Proc. Soc. Biol. Med.* **127** : 559.

Jurin, M. and Taunock, I.F. 1972. Influence of vitamin A on immunoloigcal response, *Immunology* **23** : 283-85.

Loweustein, L.M. and Lee. F. I. 1966. Hepatic cell division in aflatoxicity. *Fedn. Proc. Fedn. Am. Socs. Exp. Biol.* **25**: 2676.

Smith, R.H. 1963. The influence of toxin of *Aspergillus flavus* on the incorporation of (C_{14}) leucine into protein. *Biochem. J.* **85** : 50-51.

CHAPTER

29

NOTE ON THE EFFECTS OF AFLATOXIN ON THE TESTIS IN POULTRY

Shaik Meeera Mohiuddin

College of Veterinary Science (Andhra Pradesh Agricultural University), Tirupati, Andhra Pradesh 517 502.

The effect of graded doses of aflatoxin on the testis in growing chicks was studied, Twenty 1 day-male chicks obtained post-hatching were reared for 4 weeks. Faecal samples are blood smears were examined to rule out any possible infection. These chicks were divided into 3 groups based on their body weights, with 7 chicks in each group. Crystalline preparation of aflatoxin was dissolved in propyleneglycol to give a concentration of 100 and 200 mg per ml. Groups 1 and 2 were fed, respectively, with 100 and 200mg of aflatoxin/day/chick in proplyneglycol for 35 days. Group 3 (control), was fed with 1 ml of propyleneglycol/day/chick for 35 days. All these chicks were fed with feed manufacturer. At the end of the experimental period all the birds were sacrificed, blood was collected for estimating total RBCs, WBCs, thrombocytic and differential count, and serum for liver and testes were preserved in 10% eosin, and studied for histological changes. The right tests in all these groups were weighed. The data were analysed statistically by employing 't' test.

The haematological values did not show any differences between the groups (Table 1). The serum-alkaline phosphatase activityin birds of group 1 was not different from the values of control birds, whereas birds of group 2 showed a significant (P>0.01) increase. On autopsy the livers and testes did not show any lesions in the control group and group 1. In group 2 the livers were grossly enlarged and congested, while both the testes were markedly atrophied (P>0.01).

Livers of birds in the control group and group1 were normal histological examination, whereas those of group 2 showed congestion only. The testes of birds in control groups and group 1 were normal. The seminiferous epithelium in these tubules was arranged in a narrow column of cells, and there was evidence of spermatogeneis. In birds of group 2 developed and smaller in size than in those of group 2 and

Table 1. Haematological values, serum-alkaline phosphatase activity and testicular weights of the chicks

Treatment	PCV (%)	Hb (g%)	RBCs (million/mm³)	Thrombocytes (thousands/mm³)	WBCs (thousands/mm²)	Neutrophils (%)	Lymphocytes (%)	Monocytes (%)	Serum (*) alkaline phosphatase	Weight of testis (g)
Group 3	35.7±2.24	12.1±0.21	5.53±0.09	17.8±0.17	18.2±0.35	24.0±0.56	72.0±0.76	6.0±0.47	904.0±23.76	5.30±0.32
	(6)	(6)	(6)	(6)	(6)	(6)	(6)	(6)	(6)	(7)
Group 1	39.00±1.67	10.75±0.11	5.07±0.51	18.36±0.97	19.57±0.34	26.7±3.24	39.2±2.72	6.3±1.55	1034.7±17.6	5.210±0.37
	(6)	(6)	(6)	(6)	(6)	(6)	(6)	(6)	(6)	(7)
Group 2	38.80±0.83	12.60±0.46	4.70±1.17	17.70±1.61	25.30±1.19	73.90±1.50	1.7±0.27	1090.5±**9.93	0.35±**0.04	
(6)	(6)	(6)	(6)	(6)	(6)	(6)	(6)	(6)	(7)	

Mean ± S.E.
Figures in parentheses indicate sample size.
** . P < 0.01 ; * , mg of P/100 ml/hour.

3. They were separate wide apart from each other with large amount of connective tissues occupying in between the tubules. No histological evidence of spormatogeneis was seen.

In this study the primary effects were noticed on the germinal epithelium of testes rather than on the germinal epithelium of testes rather than of the liver. Thus it may be concluded that the germinal epithelial cells of the testes were affected earlier than the hepatic cells.

CHAPTER

30

STUDIES ON PHAGOCYTEIC ACTIVITY AND HAEMATOLOGICAL CHANGES IN AFLATOXICOSIS IN POULTRY

S..M. Mohiuddin, M. Virkram, Reddy, M. Madahva Reddy and K. Ramakrishna

Department Of Pathology, College of Veterinary Science,
Rajendranagar, Hyderabad - 500 030

Following the outbreak of Turkey 'X' disease (Blount, 1960) considerable amount of information on the aflatoxicosis has accumulated in literature. Aflatoxins are the metabolic products of the fungus *Aspergillus flavus*. The toxin are known to be hepatotoxic, teratogenic, mutogenic, carcinogenic (Legator, 1969) and antimitotic in activity (Green 1968). It also has suppressing affection immune mechanism (Mohiuddin *et al* 1981 and Pier, 1981).

In the present investigation, phagocytic activity of heterophils and Kupffer cells associated with haematoloigcal changes was investigated in aflatoxin-fed birds.

Materials and Methods

Five cockerels of about 6 months age were divided into two groups. Group 1 consisted of two cockerels which were fed with aflatoxin-free diet while Group 2 consisted of there cockerels which were fed with a diet containing aflatoxin at 20 ppm level. The fungus *A. flavus* was grown on maize which contained mainly aflatoxin B1 and was used in this experiment. These two groups were maintained over a period of three months and were inoculated with 1 ml. of saturated carbon solution i/v, using wing vein. After 48 hours, they were sacrificed, blood was collected.

The slight increase in total WBC counts, mainly consisting of heterophiles suggests the effect of eliciting inflammatory response. However, the phagocytic activity of hetrophilies in toxin-fed birds appeared less when compared to control birds. Michael *et al* (1973) reported the dietary aflatoxin at 1.35 mg/g and 5mg/g of feed

Haematological and heterophilic phagocytic activity

PCV	Hb gm %	Total RBC count	Thrombocytic count	Total basophilic count	Total WBC count	Heterophiles	Lymphos %	Eosin %	Mono %	Base %	Heterophilic activity +ve	Phagocytic -ve	
Control group													
1.	26.0	7.3	2.40	21,400	2,525	18,250	48.0	2.0	2.0	2.0	95	5	
2.	28.0	7.5	2.50	21,600	2,650	18,500	47.0	45.0	3.0	3.0	3.0	92	8
Total	54.0	14.8	4.90	43,000	5,170	36,850	95.0	91.0	5.0	5.0	4.0	187	13
Meal	27.0	7.4	2.45	21,500	2,585	47.5	45.5	2.5	2.5	2.0	94	6	
Aflatoxin-fed groups													
1.	25.0	6.3	1.40	14,250	1,225	20,550	67.0	26.0	4.0	1.0	2.0	80	20
2.	26.0	6.2	1.50	14,550	1,525	20,450	61.0	31.0	2.0	2.4	4.0	85	15
3.	25.0	604	1.55	15,050	1,350	20,600	68.8	30.0	1.0	1.0	-	87	13
Total	76.0	18.9	4.45	43,850	61,600	4196.0	87.0	7.0	4.0	6.0	252	48	
Mean	25.3	6.3	1.48	14,613	1,366	20,533	54.3	29.0	2.3	1.3	2.0	84	16

significantly decreased the clearance of colloidal carbon from circulation by the reticuloendothelial system of the chicks. A decrease ($P<0.5$) in phagocytic activity of thrombocytes and circulating monocytes was recorded when chicks were fed with aflatoxin at 5 or 10mg/g. Feed (Chang Hamilton 1979a) and at 2.5 mg/g of feed and above (Chang and Hamilton 1979b) respectively. In these studies, a decreased phagocytic activity off reticuloendothelial system and circulating monocytes was noted in the birds fed with aflatoxin at a level of 25 ppm for a periof of 3 weeks. The phagocytic activity of heterophilic and Kupffer cells was reduced in the present investigation when these birds were fed at 20 ppm, of aflatoxin a smaller dose level over a period of 12 weeks. Though there is increase in heterophilic count the accompanying effect of lymphopaenia points out at the suppressing action of aflatoxin on immunological system as the lymphocytes are the main cells concerned with humoral and cell mediated immunity. The lymphopaenia observed in the toxin-fed birds further supports the earlier observations made by Giambrone *et al* (1978) and Mohiuddin *et al* (1981) and Pier (1981) regarding the suppressive effect of aflatoxin on antibody synthesis.

The main histogical changes observed in the liver of aflatoxin-fed birds were, periportal fatty changes (Fig. 1) and the loss of normal hepatic architecture. Though Kupffer cells are prominent, they did not show the presence of carbon particles. The Kupffer cells in the control birds were not prominent but deposition of carbon particles (Fig. 2). The perioportal fatty changes and necrosis in the liver and hypetrophied Kupffer cells are suggestive of aflatoxicosis.

Summary

The effect of aflatoxicosis on phagocytic activity and haemotological changes were studied in birds. These birds were fed aflatoxin 20 ppm in the feed over a period of three months. The phagocytic activity of heterophiles and Kupffer cells and determined by injecting 1 ml of saturated solution of carbon. The results indicated that aflatoxin has a depressing effect on the phagocytie activity of heterophiles and Kupffer cells also lowers haematological values. The total basophilic and thrombocytic counts were found decreased in aflatoxin-fed birds suggesting that aflatoxin lowers the resistance of the body to infection.

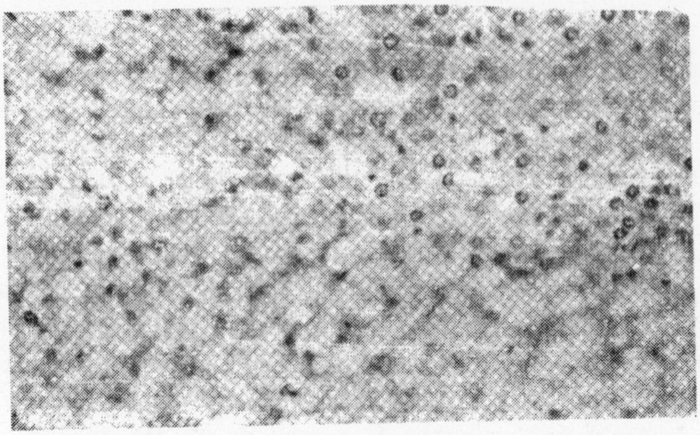

Fig.1. Liver showing periportal fatty changes. Kupffer cells did not contain coal particles.

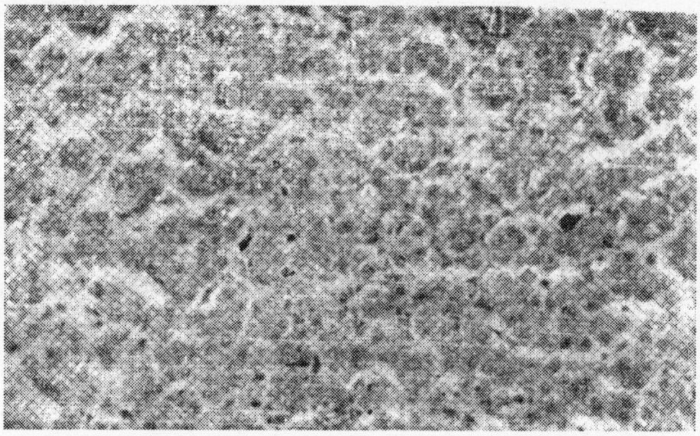

Fig.2. Kupffer cells are loaded with coal particles.

ACKNOWLEDGEMENT

The authors are thankful to Dr. R.R. Reddy, Principal, College of Veterinary Science for his encuragement in carrying out of this investigation.

REFERENCES

Blount. L.P. (1960) *J. Br. Turkey Fd. 9 : 52*

Chand, N. and Eyre, F. (1978) *Avian Diseases 22 : 639.*

Chang, C.F. and Hamilton, P.B. (1979a) *Poult. Sci.* **58** *: 559*

– – – – (1979b) *Ibid* **58** *: 562*

Giambrone, J.J. Ewert, D.L., Wyatt, P.D. *Am. J. vet. Res.* **39** *305.*

Green, S. (1968) *Nature* **220** *: 931*

Legator, W.P. (1969) J. Am. Vet. Med. Ass. **155** : 2080.

Michael, G.Y., Thaxton. P. and Hamilton, P.B. (1973) *Poult. Sci.* **52 :** 1206.

Mohiuddin, S.M., Mhendranath, M. and Yadagiri, B, (1081) *Indian J. Anim, Sci.* **51** : 77.

Pier, A.C. (1981) *Adv. vet. Sci. Comp. Med.* **25** : 185.

CHAPTER

31

EFFECT OF DIETARY AFLATOXIN ON THE DEVELOPMENT OF IMMUNITY AGAINST NEWCASTLE DISEASE VIRUS IN CHICKEN

A. Nageswara Rao, V. Ravindra A. Reddy, P. V. Rao, B.J. Sharma and S.M. Mohiuddin
Andhra Pradesh Agricultural University, Hyderabad, Andhra Pradesh *500030.*

The present study was aimed primarily to evaluate the effect of dietary aflatoxin on immune response against Newcastle (Ranikhet) disease virus in commerical White Leghorn (WL) male chicks. In addition, the effect of dietary aflatoxin on leukocyte counts, serum protein and growth and histopathology of immunerelated organs was studied.

Two experiments with a3 x 2 factorail design were conducted with diets containing 3 levels aflatoxin (corresponding to 0, 0.5 and 1.0 ppm B_1 activity) fed to 2 groups of commercial day-old WL male chicks, one vaccinated and the other unvaccinated against Newcastle disease. The vaccinated group had immunization scheduled on 8th day (F_1), 9th week (RB) in experiment 2. The duration of experiment 1 was 0-18 weeks with 80 chicks per treatment and of experiment 2 was 0-9 weeks with 12 chicks per treatment of uniform body weight at day-old age.

Blood samples were collected at weekly intervals from all the 12 birds in each treatment group once before vaccination and 4 times after vaccination for the evaluation of humoral (HI titres) and cell-mediated immunity (LMIT). In addition, body-weight gain was recorded, at end of experiment, 1, blood samples taken from wing vein from 4 birds per treatment were used to study the total and differential leukocyte counts. Gross and histopathology of immune-related organs, viz. bursa of Farbicius, thymus and spleen preserved in 10% buffered formalin, were studied in 6 birds per treatment by slaughtering them at 12th and 18th weeks age in experiment 1. The data of various parameters were analysed, statistically (Snedecor and Cochran, 1968). The data of total leukocyte count and HI titres were subjected to logarithmic transformation before analysis.

Body weights and organ weights

Body weights of chicken for 0-18 weeks decreased ($P<0.01$) due to feeding of aflatoxin from 0.5 ppm onwards (Table 1) as was observed by Rajesekhara Reddy *et al.* (1982). At 1.0 ppm level of dietary aflatoxin the spleen was enlarged and the bursa regressed (Table 1). The bursal regression was significant ($P>0.05$) old but not when 18 weeks old. Since the bursa normally gains the maximum size by 9-10 weeks followed by a gradual regression thereafter, the absence of a significant effect in bursal weight at 18th week with or without the toxin feeding might be a consequence of natural regression of the bursa. The thymus weight was, however, not influenced by toxin levels tested either at 12th or 18th week of age (Table 1). A similar thymus response was observed by Thazton *et al.* (1974) at comparable levels of toxin feeding. Serum proteins decreased with each increase in aflatoxin level from 0.5 ppm onwards. This was again in conformity with our earlier reports wherein also serum proteins were lowered from 0.25 ppm onwards (Rajesekhara Reddy *et al.*,1982). In this study neither total leukocyte count nor the differential leukocyte count were affected by the aflatoxin levels tested. Tung *et al.* (1975) made similar observations up to 2.5 ppm, but at a higher dose (10 mg/g) the total leukocyte count was about 3 times that of control.

Humoral immunity

The humoral immunity was affected significantly due to 1.0 ppm dietary aflatoxin (Table 2), Chenchev *et al.* (1978), Mohiudin *et al.* (1981) and Boulton *et al.* (1982). Observed poor immune responses against ND vaccination even with lower dietary aflatoxin levels ranging from 0.2 to 0.64 ppm. The adverse effect of alfatoxin on humoral immunity was consistent only after primary vaccination but was negated after booster vaccination. This observation supports the Boulton *et al.* (1983).

Table 1. Body weight and organ weights of chicken as influenced by dietary aflatoxin level at 18 weeks of age

Age (weeks)		Aflatoxin (ppm)		
		0	0.5	1.0
Weight gain (kg)	18	1.426[a]	1.314[b]	1.258[b]
Bursal weight (g/100)	12	0.39[a]	0.32[ab]	0.25[b]
(g body wt)	18	0.17	0.13	0.13
Thymus weight	12	0.48	0.41	0.37
(g/100 g body wt)	18	0.40	0.34	0.32
Spleen weight	12	0.18	0.21B	0.23B
(g/100 g body wt)	18	0.16P	0.19PQ	0.22Q
Serum proteins (g/100 ml)	18	5.7[a]	5.3[b]	4.8[a]

Means bearing the same capital letter superscripts (P<001) or the small letter superscripts (P<0.05) do not differ significantly.

Cell-mediated immunity

The cell-mediated immunity, as measured by LMIT though significantly (P<0.01) increased by vaccination, was not influenced by the aflatoxin at any of the levels tested in either of the experiments (Table 3). Giambrone *et al.*(1978) found a deficient cell-mediate immunity in chicken fed a high level of aflatoxin (2.5 mg/g).

Histopathlogy

Occasional areas of lmyphoid depletion in follicles of spleen and bursa of Fabricious observed confirm the reports by giambrone *et al.* (1978). However, the lymphoid depletion in the thymus observed by Giambrone *et al.* (1978) was not evident in this study, possible due to the very high levels (2.5 mg/g) of aflatoxin used by them. Histopathological changes in the bursa of Fabricius brought about by aflatoxin in were similar to those reported by Rajesekhara Reddy *et*

Table 3. CMI response expressed in terms of per cent area of

Table 2. Humoral immune response in terms of HI titres (log 10) against ND virus in chicken fed different level of aflatoxin

Dietary aflatoxin (ppm)	After primary (RB) vaccination at 9th week of age					After booster (RB) vaccination at 15th week of age				Combined mean
	Ist week	2nd week	3rd week	4th week	Mean	Ist week	2nd week	3rd week	Mean	
					Experiment 1					
0	1.94	2.08	2.10	1.92	2.01a	2.15	2.27	2.20	2.21	2.11A
0.5	1.78	2.00	1.93	1.70	1.87[ab]	2.10	2.20	2.10	2.13	1.99AB
1.0	1.65	1.86	1.83	1.74b	1.74[b]	2.08	2.12	2.05	2.14	1.90
					Experiment 2					
	After primary (F^1) vaccination at eighth day of age					After booster (BR) vaccination at 6 weeks of age				
0	1.48	1.60	1.63	1.54	1.56[a]	2.08	2.00	1.95	2.01	1.79[A]
0.5	1.54	1.57	1.51	1.44	1.52[a]	2.04	2.00	1.93	1.99	1.76[A]
1.0	1.30	1.44	1.35	1.30	1.35[ab]	1.94	1.90	4.74	1.86	1.61[B]

Table 3. CMI response expressed in terms of per cent area of migration's of leukocytes as influenced by dietary aflatoxin.

Dietary aflatoxin (ppm)		Prevaccinations	After primary (RB) vaccinations (mean for 4 weeks)	After booster (RB) vaccinations (mean for 3 weeks)	Combined (mean)
			Experiment 1		
0	UV[1]	100.0	100.7^{A}	99.4^{A}	100.1^{a}
	V[2]	97.6	83.7^{B}	83.4^{B}	85.6^{b}
0.5	UV	99.8	99.4^{A}	99.4^{A}	99.6^{a}
	V	99.8	85.5^{B}	85.5^{B}	87.5^{b}
1.0	UV	98.7	99.7^{A}	99.7^{A}	99.5^{a}
	V	99.8	86.7^{B}	86.7^{B}	87.9^{b}
			Experiment 2 *After (F[1]) vaccination*		
0	UV	101.1	100.8^{A}	99.8^{A}	100.3^{a}
	V	102.2	93.7^{B}	85.5^{B}	89.1^{b}
0.5	UV	101.1	99.8^{A}	100.7^{A}	100.1^{a}
	V	102.2	93.6^{B}	86.2^{B}	89.9^{b}
1.0	UV	101.1	100.1^{A}	99.7^{A}	99.9^{a}
	V	102.2	93.4^{B}	88.1^{A}	90.7^{b}

UV[1], Unvaccinated; V[2], Vaccinated.
Means bearing same capital ($P<0.05$) or small ($P<0.005$) letter superscripts do not differ significantly.

migrations of leukocytes as influencd by dietary aflatoxin

It was concluded that humoral immune response of chicken against ND virus and that too only after primary vaccination was adversely affected by feeding aflatoxin-infested diets from 1.0 ppm onwards. However, the LMIT, thymus weight, total and differential leukocyte counts were not influenced by toxin levels tested.

REFERENCES

Boulton, S. L., Dick, J. W. and Hughes, B.L. 1982. Effect of dietary aflatoxin and ammonia-inactivated aflatoxin on Newcastle disease antibody titres in layer breeders. *Avian Diseases* **36** : 1-6.

Chenchev, L., Kosnov. G. Alexandrov, A., Parlov, N., and Kovacheva., K. 1978. Effect of afflatoxin on the serum profile and antibody production in fowls. *Veterinarnomedit sinski Nauki* **15** : 47-51.(*fide Poultry Abstracts* **5** : 2857.)

Giambrone, J.J., Ewert, D.L., Wyatt, R.D. and Edison, C.S. 1978. Effect of alfatoxin on the humoral an cell-mediated immune systems of the chickens. *Amercina Journal of Veterinary Research* **39** : 305-308.

Mohiuddin, S.M., Mahendranath, D., Yadgiri, B. and Ahmed, S.R., 1981. Studies on the effect of aflatoxin on antibody synthesis against Ranikhet disease vaccine in chicks, *Indian Journal of Animal Sciences* : **51** 77-82.

Rajesekhara Reddy, A., Reddy, V.R., Rao, P.V. and Yadgiri, B. 1982. Studies on the effect of dietary aflatoxin on the heamatology and performance of commercial broiler chicks. *Indian Journal of Animal Sciences* **52** : 405-410.

Snedecor, G.W. and Cochran, W.G 1968. *Statistical Methods.* 6th edn. Oxford and IBH Publishing Co., Calcutta.

Thaxton, J.P. Tung, H.T. and Hamilton, P.B. 1974. Immunosuppression in chickens by aflatoxin. *Poultry Science* **53** : 721-25.

Tung, H.T., Cook. F.W., Wyatt, R.D and Hamilton, P.B. 1975. The anemia caused by aflatoxin. *Poultry Science* **54** : 1962-69.

CHAPTER 32

NUTRITION MYCOTOXICOSIS AND ITS CONTROL

Dr. S.M. Mohiuddin
Professor and Head, Department of Pathology, College of Veterinary Science, Rajendranagar, Hyderabad 500 030.

Mycotoxin are defined as fungal metabolites produced in feedstuffs which can cause disease and death in man and animals. There is now a growing awareness of the implications of mycotoxins as frequent contaminants of agricultural commodities and their associated health and economic hazards. There are over 300 fungi known to produce the mycotoxins. We know very little about the toxicity they produce, excepting a few toxins. The important mycotoxins identified are aflatoxins, mycotoxins, trichothecense, citrinin and zearalenone. These toxic agents are ubiquitous in distribution and have been isolated from a wide variety of foods and mixed feeds.

Contamination of feed

About 100 fungi that grow on standing crops or stored feeds are known to produce toxic substances and about 20 of these substances have been associated with harvesting, naturally -occuring diseases in man and animals. In majority of the cases the fungal contamination occurs during Improper storage of feed ingredients and mixed feeds can lead to them being contaminated with fungi. Many fungi are opportunistic pathogens which can invade and produce mycotoxin when the grains are in the field.

A moisture content of 12% of and above in the feed, relative humidity of 80-90%, and temperature ranging from 10°C to 42°C is sufficient for prolific fungal growth. All these condition are available in tropical countries like India.

Many of the mycotoxins are heat-stable and survive pelleting and other processing operations. Mycotoxins are also nonantigenic. Except aflatoxins, very little information is available regarding pathogenesis, or clinical effects or acute and chronic affects of these toxins and diagnosis.

Effects of Mycotoxins

Among the various mycotoxins, aflatoxins are considered to be the most potent and harmful. Aflatoxin are the metabolic products of the fungi Aspergillus Flavus and Aspergillus are the metabolic products of the fungi Aspergillus Flavus and Aspergillus Parasiticus. They produce aflatoxins B1, B2, G1, G2, M1 and M2. Among these aflatoxin B1 is highly toxic and harmful.

Aflatoxins are primarily hepatotoxic, secondary Carcinogenic. Tetrogenic and Mustogenic. Effects on poultry production are

1. Reduce body weight gain.
2. Decrease egg production as well as egg weight.
3 Suppress the immune-system, making them highly susceptible to diseases.
4. Disrupt bone development causing ricketic type problems.
5. Induce many nutritional problems through effects on nutrient absorption and metabolism.
6. Cause bruises in broilers resulting in condemnation of the carcass.
7. Lowest hatchability and increase in embryonic mortality.
8. Economic effects of Mycotoxins and Aflatoxins on poultry Reduced rate of egg production.

In another study at the National Institute of Nutrition, Hyderababad, it was found that feeding of 0.7 PPM of aflatoxin-contaminated feed for a short duration had resulted in over 30% reduction in egg production. Loss of Rs. 45, 000 occurred over a three week period in a farm with 11,000 layers. Another mycotoxin, mycotoxin is primarily a nephrotoxin in poultry. Ochratoxin is three times more toxic to broiler chicken than aflatoxin. T-2 toxin is redosmetic toxin and its action is similar to radiation.

Mycotoxin Interactions

Several analytical laboratories have found that most mycotoxin contaminated samples contain more than just a single mycotoxin. When aflatoxin and orchatoxin co-contaminates of poultry feed they interact in a synergistic manner. The toxicity that results from dual exposure to aflatoxin and ochratoxin is more severe than the sum of the individual toxicity of these mycotoxins. This may be one reason why very low levels of aflatoxin in the field could produce significant ill effects in poultry compared to laboratory studies where only a single mycotoxin is studied. Due to interaction the symptoms are also different. The target organ of the interaction between aflatoxin and ochratoxin and citrinin can be characterised an antagonistic. Even though the interaction is antagonist, the animals compared to growing much poorly in the interaction group when compared to growing animals on just a single toxin. The mycotoxin combinationof aflatoxin and T02 toxin is found to exhibit a synergistic effect.

Mycotoxin safe limits

Opinion is ananimous as far as the effects of aflatoxin on poultry production can concerned. However, as far as the tolerable level of aflatoxin is concerned, there is total diversity of opinion. Levels raining from 20 ppm to 2000 ppm have been sounded about as "safe" level. One of the reasons for each such wide ranging claim is that many studies have taken mortality as the criterion for defining safe limits. However, in poultry farming is not enough to just keep the birds alive without production, which matters, more.

The European Economic Community (EEC) limit of 20 ppb (incorporated into the legislation of all member states) assumes significance. While it may be argued that this limit is not totally applicable to Indian conditions, what is significant is that this limit was fixed keeping in view two well defined parameters that the allowed levels for aflatoxins should not.

1. Impair the health of animals and hence us periodicity.
2. Be sufficient to enter the human food chanvia animal products. To determine the relative safety of feed, misused on single mycotoxin analysis may grossly underestimate the true risk wearer taking.

Many factors are found to affect the toxicity to aflatoxins are these include (a) genetic variability (b) nutritional status of animal (c) environmental stress, and (d) sex differences.

Thus, safety is concept that usually based on the individual's limited experience. It had been stressed that there can be no safe level of mycotoxin, as even very minute doses over a prolonged period may prove to be carcinogenic.

Aflatoxin levels:

Data on Aflatoxins levels analysed in different feed ingredients, from June 1988 to March 1990.

Sr. No	Samples	Samples analysed	Aflatoxin +ve	Toxin levels ppm
1.	Compound feed	211	102	0.02-0.4
2.	G.N. cake	169	94	0.01-0.3
2.	Fish	32	10	0.01-0.2
4.	Maize	41	11	0.01-0.1
5.	Liver Meat	9	9	0.01-0.3
6.	Meat Meal	2	2	0.4
7.	Bajra	7	3	0.10-0.2
8.	Soyabean meat	5	4	0.10-0.2
9.	Dal cake	2	2	Below 0.05
10.	Sunflower cake	2	2	0.10-0.2

Methods to prevent mycotoxicosis:

Mycotoxicosis is a global problem that is very difficult to tackle. The control method tried include the following.

1. Establishing a mycotoxin-screening programme.
2. Careful monitoring and controlling of the moisture level of feed ingredient.
3. Periodically cleaning all feed handling equipment with a 5% to 10% beaching solution.
4. Keeping the time from manufacture of feeds to presentation to the animals at a minimum.
5. Minimising pellet breakdown to reduce the level of fineness in the feed.
6. Using a mould-inhibitor to prevent further contamination of feed ingredients and mixed feeds.
7. Using fed-additives to reduce the toxicity of aflatoxins.
8. Detoxification inactivation of mycotoxin-contaminated food and feed have been proposed.

They are (a) the ammoniation of grains and feedstuffs to destroy aflatoxins and (b) the addition of "sorbent" to the grains and feedstuffs to destroy the aflatoxin.

In condition, mycotoxins have been recognised as significant economic and health hazards on a worldwide scale. A concerned inter-disciplinary research effort involving the acadèmic, government and industrial agencies, to develop viable measures to solve this important problem is clearly warranted at this this juncture.

CHAPTER 33

PATHOLOGY OF FOOD-BORNE MYCOTOXINS IN POULTRY

Dr. S.M. Mohiuddin and Dr. R. Sreenath Reddy
Department of Pathology Veterinary College, Rajendranagar, Hyderabad - 500 030

INTRODUCTION

Mycotoxins, a group of metabolites elaborated by fungi, in the media in which they grow, are of great significance in the health of animals than we realize. Although many species of fungi are common in feeds only few fungis responsible to produce potent toxins have been identified. They are aflatoxin produced by *Aspergillus flavus;* Zearalenone, produced by *Aspergillus ochracens,* produced by P. *citrinum and* sterigmatocystin produced by *Aspergillus versicolar.*

Aspergillus versicolor

Ingestion of these mycotoxin contaminated feeds can lead to various clinical and subclinical manifestations. Mycotoxins has affected the health of birds when consumed the infected feed thus affecting the poultry industry. The various manifestations of mycotoxicosis are low nitrogen, low metabolic utilization of consumed feed, poor aflatoxin alters the cellular integrity of the host (Doerr *et al.* 1978) and predisposes the birds to microbial and other diseases (Wong and Hsieh, 1980).

Tapia *et al.* (1980) reported the presence of enlarged and pale liver, with severe degenetive lesions and proliferation and hepatocytes in the periportal region.

A hypocarotenoidaemia and hepatic heperlipaemia were seen during chronic aflatoxicosis in broiler chicks (Doerr *et al.*, 1983).

Moorthy *et al.* (1985) observed hepatic lesions in chickens given 6.25 ppm 3.12 ppm aflatoxin in feed. Important gross lesions included pale yellow livers with haemorrhages, haematomas and nodules. Important histological findings included lipidosis, sinusoid congestion, periavascular haemorrhages, bileduct hyperplasia, phlebitis and veno-occlusive lesions.

B. Ochratoxin

Ochratoxins are the most widely recognized toxins produced by *A. ochraceus A. culture* of *Aspergillus ochraceus* grown on crushed moist wheat for 20 days at 20°C gives a high moist wheat for 20 days at 20°C give a high yield of ochratoxins. Extraction of the toxins is by methods similar to those used in the extraction in aflatoxins.

Optimum production of ochratoxin on maize, rice or wheat occurs at 28°C after 6.14 days; depending on the substrate. The toxin is stable and withstands autoclaving for a period of 3 hrs. A pH of 6.0-6.3 is recommended for production media.

The LD 50 of ochralopin is for one-day-old ducklings is 25 ug and for chickens it is 216 ug. Ochratoxin is the most toxic among all the metabolites.

Aspergillus ochracens

Dchratoxins affect many animals and cause death in the chickens also. In 14 week old WLH chickens, ochratoxin causes a retarding of sexual maturity and feeble egg production at low concentration and at higher concentrations a very low egg production with hepatic and renal disorders.

Threon *et al.* (1964) investigated the histopathology of ochratoxicosis in ducklings and reported an increase in fatty vacuolation, changes in the matrix of the mitochondria, and disorganization of the endoplasmic reticulum of hepatosities.

Doupnik and Peckham (1970) and Peckam *et al* (1970) studied ochratoxicosis in young WLH cockerels and reported postmortem findings of dehydration, emaciation, altered mucosal linings of the gizzard, few small haemorrhages in the prventriculus and enteritis while the main gross findings was visceral gout. Microscopically they found acute nephrosis, heaptic degeneration and suppression of hematopoiesis in descending order of frequency.

Tucker and Hamilton (1971) reported ochratoxin to cause pathological changes in chickens such as emaciation, altered linings of the gizzard and increased liver glycogen.

Huff *et al.* (1974) studied ochratoxicosis in broiler chicken and reported enlarged kidney, crop, proventiculus, gizzard and liver, while the bursa fabricius were segressed, Enlarged kidneys and reduced growth rates are most sensitive indicators. They also reported the following gross pathological lesions-petichae of the papillage of proventriculus, slight grizzard erosions and paleness of the kidney, liver and pancrease.

Huff *et al.* (1975) reported that ochratoxin induces enlarged kidneys, impaired real function, increased uric acid production and concluded that ochratoxin is a severe nephroxin in young broiler chickens.

Chang *et al.* (1979) reported that ochratoxin-A induced a severe leucocytopenia (primarily) and monocytopenia to a lesser extent and implied that functioning of the immune system might be affected.

Ochratoxin-A induces impaired phagocytic ability of heterophils (Chang and Hamilton, 1980) and thymus regression in broiler chicken (Chang *et al.*, 1981).

Hamilton *et al.* (1982) observed an increased incidence of air-sacculitis in several field outbreak of ochratoxicos in broier fowls and related it to the possible imunisuppressive effects of the mycotxin.

In young broiler chicks, ochratoxin A caused a significant enlargement of the kidney, liver and proventiriculus, whereas the thymus and the bursa of fabricius were reduced in size. It principally affected the proximal conveluted trubriles of the kidney causing severe distention, enlargement and hypertrophy resulting in thickening of the glomerular basement membrane. In the liver vacuolation and glycogen accumulation of in the hepatocytes, also regression of the lymphoid cells population in the imunoloigcal organs (Dwivedi and Burns, 1984).

Dwivedi *et al.* (1984) reported the following ultrastructural changes in the liver and kidney in ochratoxicosis-A in young broiler chicks. There was increased accumulation of cytoplasm glycogen in the hepatocytes, abnormal mitochondrial ring formation in kidneys. Identical findings were also reported by Burns and Dwivedi (1986).

Ochration A caused a significant depression in immunoglobin containing cells in all the lymphoid organ studied. (Dwivedi and Burns, (1984).

Bodnanhuke and Kasprok (1984) reported the presence of haemorrhages in various tissues and catarrhal gastritis and enteritis.

Feeding ochratoxin A from 0 to 21 days of age was associated with proximul tubular intranclear membrane bound inclusion, elongated tortuous and ring-shaped mitchondria, enlarged mitochrondrial metric granules with hyaline centres and an increase in size and membrane of peroxisomes and secondary lyposomes (Bronw *et al.*1986).

C. Citrinin

Citrinin is an important toxin production of which is mainly associated with *Pencillium citrinum* and related species. This species has been frequently isolated from mouldy groundnuts. It forms grey green colories which becomes grey, or olive green, as the spores mature, in the media.

Citrinin can be isolated by treating on alcoholic extract of moulded rice with benzene and ether. Citrinin remains in the alcoholic fraction.

Citrinin is essentially a toxin of live and the kidneys, and is particularly responsible for kidney lesions in which there is considerable enlargement of the collecting tabules. It is though to act by destroying the epithlium of the tabules and subsequent diffused formation of the connective tissues (interesting fibrosis) has been reported. Exclation of urine is upto 2 and 2½ times greater than normal.

Carlton (1980) noted that principle histological lesions are seen in the kidney and the nephrotoxic effects of citrinin were considered he prinicipal cause of death.

Histopathological alteration were most prominent in the kidneys which includes degeneration and necrosis of tubular epithelia cells of both the proximal and distal convulted tubules. Hepatic lesion wares multiple foci of necrosis and haemorragic lymphoid necrosis depletion were found in the bursa of fabricius, thymus, caecal tonsil and spleen in birds (Mehdi *et al.*, 1981).

Mehdi *et al.*, (1983) observered that the mycotoxin was nephrotic and renal lesions were more severe in tukeys than ducklings; and were characterized by degeneration and necrosis of renal tubular epithelium. Further were also noted in liver. Similar findings were also reported by Mehdi *et al.* (1984).

Hinatow and Wideman (1985) reported that cirrinin acts directly on the kidneys to alter several tubular directly on the alter several tublar transport processes. These include increase urinary flaourate free water clearance and in sodium potassium and imorganic phosphate excretion.

Feeding citrinin from 1 to 21 days of age was associated with proximal tubular nuclear incusions, elongated tortuous and ring-shaped mitochondria and an increase in size and number of perosisomes and secondary lysosomes (Brown *et al.*, 1986).

D. Sterigmatocystin

Toxicoses which involve *A. versocolor* are probably due to sterigmatocystin, and related metabolites, which it products. Sterigmatocoystin itself is a pale yellow crystalin compound, which is isoluable in water.

A practical method of analysing sterigmatocystin in grain and oilseeds has been described by vorster and Purshase. It is based on the conversion of this metabolite into a monoacetate which is much more fluoresent.

Sterignatocystin, at doses varyingfrom 19-100 mg/kg cause lvier nerosis which may be either centrolobular (when adm, orally) or periportal (when adm. I/P). When the doses is very high (144 mg/kg) haemorrhages and severe necrosis of the tubules and glomerules of the kidney are seen.

Sterigmatocystin is metabolized and secreted within 12-24 hrs in the urine, faeces and especially in the Gastrointestinal tract of chicken.

Histopatholoigcal changes in the livers of ducklings fed sterigmatocystin produced by *A. versicolor* was studied. Haemorrhages, hepatic parenchymal degeneration and necrosis fatty changes, fibroblast proliferation and mitotic figures of the bileduct cells were observed (Yoon, 1983).

Gross and histological examination revealed rapturned egg follicles, swollen kidney with dilated tubules and hemorrhages, petechial haemorrhages in the fatty tissue and degenerative changes in the nuclei of hepatocytes (Pojanvirta *et al.*, 1984).

Ivanokakii (1986) observedon postmortem hepatic degeneration, catasrrhal enteritis and sub-capsular haemorrhages in kidneys, when this mycotoxin was given varying from 40-400 mg/kg BW.

E. Z. Earlenone

Fusarium graminearum is the principle organism which produces Zearalenone. The mould is frequently seen on rye, oats, barley and rarely in rice. The infection of barley may be detected by descoloration of the spikelet which becomes yellowish and then brownish. Sometimes a red eflorscence of mycelium is visible of the surface.

A good yield of zearlalenon can be obtained on maize, containing atleast 45% water, or on rice at 12°C. At 25°C the toxin production is nil, and moreover, a preliminary passage at a low temperature seems to be necessary to obtain any yield at temperature greater than 12°C.

The symptoms of toxicity incldue mainly disorder fo the digestive tract accompanied by diarrhoea, often with blood faeces. There is weight loss, and a general loss of appetite. Frequent haemorhagic lesions are also noted in the stomach, the heart, the intestines and lungs.

When turkey poults were fed a diet containing 300 ppm zearalenone or a diet composed of fusarium invaded corn at a level of 10%, swelling of the vent, mucos secretion, and cystine, development in the cloaca occured (Meronuck *et al.* 1970).

Speers *et al.* (1970) reported that the feeding of zearalenone or fusarium invaded corn (300 to 1600 ppm) to 10 day old WLH chicks did not cause nay prominent signs except for an increase in weight gainand high incidence of cystine development in the genital tract.

Possibilities and Limitations of Diagnosis

The treatment and control of cycotoxicosis to be of optimum value, the diagnosis must be as accurate as possible, since in general, there are two ways of making diagnosis. The first method is based on past experience and depends upon the recognition for the syndromes. The second method is diagnosis by reasoning and is based on a rational summing up of the clinical and laboratory findings and progression by logical steps to a final diagnosis. In practice the first method is often used and a experience is enlarged which becomes reasonably accurate in many cases. However its weakness lies in the fact that so few cases are identical and many will be seen that ar sufficiently atypical to make the use of the method highly inaccurate. As a general rule, diagnosis by reasoning is the method of choice and the following description, provides a useful framework for its development.

General physical Ex: for detection of clinically significant abnormalities. Determines Abnormalities of function present.

Special Ex: of suspect systems of organs, physical and laboratory. Determines system or organ involved or body as a whole

Special Ex: of identical system. Ex: exploratory laboraotory, endoscopy Determines location of lesion in the suptem or organ.

Speical Ez: of lesion eg: biopsy, response of treatment, examination of Fluids. Determines Type of lesion

Special ex: of Specimens eg: blood, urine, feed or soil samples, by chemical microbiological & parasitological means. Determines specific cause of lesion.

SUMMARY

The presence of mycotoxin, in feed induces a series of pathological changes which sometimes even led to death. The various pathological findings of the different authors has been simmarised and given below.

A. Aflatoxins

Contrary to the situation in mammals, the liver of poultry suffering aflatoxicosis doesn't show fibrosis. Degeneation of the cells of the hepatic parecnchyma is particularly noticeable accompanied by the active regeneration by proliferation of the epithelium of the bile ducts from the periportal regions. Haemorrhages could be observed on the heart, kidneys, lungs, pancreas and spleen. Liver had nodular growths of varying size of 1-3 mm in diameter. Microscopic changes of the liver revealed congestion in the sinusoids haemorrages at one end of the vessels giving 'paravacular' type of distribution besides bile duct hyperplasia.

Sclerosis of the spleenic, corronayr, renal and pulmonary vessels was observed uniformly. Chronic bronchitis, with hypertrophy of bronchial epithelium and submucosal lymphoidal infiltration was seen occasionally. Kidney revealed coboida changed in cells lining the glomerular tufts: mild periglomerular fibrosis; crowding of the glomeruli and cystic changes in the tubules.

In the ducklings, a single dose of aflatoxin is sufficient to obtain a rapid proliferation which reaches its maximum after 3 days. Associated with this there is degernation of peripheral parenchymatous cells. This lesion rapidly regresses after Ten days, some accumulation of basophilic cells is observed and in some regions, it is very difficult to distinguish regenerating basophils from parenchymatous cells. In chronic cases, the liver is enlarged and shows a brown or greenish colour; the surface has irregular granulations sometimes forming into large nuduels. The parenchymatus cells are inflated and cytoplasm is granular and eosionophilic; few cells show necrosis, the nuclei are inflated and hyperhcrnomatic, hyperplasia of the bile duct is already clear at this stage and the egg shaped cells appear radially dispoersed from the peripartal zone. After 2 weeks there is a considerable hyperplasia of the bile ducts After 3 weeks hepatic nodubles, with hyperplastic cells are separated by bands of bileducts epithelium.

Kidneys are swollen and pale brown. Protein debris is present in abnormal quanitities in the dilated tubules and large nuclei with strange morphology are visible in some of the degenerated epithelial cells.

It may be noted that the enlargement of the hepatic cells (megalocytosis) and swelling of the nuclei (Karyomegaly) are seen in cattle, ducks and turkeys, whereas is chickens, swelling of the nucleus without megalocytosis may be seen.

B. Ochratoxin

Salient pathological findings of ochratoxicosis in chickens are given below:

(a) Renal disorders are tubular necrosis of the kidneys which includes significant enlargement of the kidneys, severe distension and enlargement and hypertrophy of proximal and convulited tubules, thickening of the glomercular basement membranes.

(b) Hepatic disorders and necrosis of peioportal cells in the liver which is generally associated with isolated cells and rorely with large group, just as with aflatoxicosis fatty Infilatration of the liver cells is observed but there is no proliferation of bile ducts.

(c) A few reports of the effects of ochratoxicosis and on the immunology of birds includes.

1. Lymphoid cell depletion in the bursa of fabricius.
2. Thymus regression.
3. Imparied phagocytic ability of heterophils.
4. Leucopenia.

(d) Ochratoxin feeding results in increased incidence of air sacculitis.

(e) Histopatholoigal changes include increase in fatty vacuolation, changes in the matirix of the mitochronidria and disorganization of the endoplasm of hepatosites.

C. Citrinin

Principal pathological lesions of citrinin toxicity are seen in kidney and liver were considered to the principle cause of death.

In the kidneys, degeneration and recrosis of tubular epithelial cells of both the proximal and converted tubules are seen. Hepatic lesion were multiple foci of necrosis and depletion were found in the vursa of fabricius, thymus, caecal tonsil and spleen in birds.

Citrnin is thought to act by destroying the epithelium of the tables and a susbsequent diffuse formation of the connective tissues (interestitial fibrosis) has also been reported.

D. Sterigmatocystin

Sterigmatocystin at doses varying from 18-100 mg/kg causis liver necrosis which may be either centrilobular or periportal. When the doses is high, haemorrhages and severe necrosis of the tubules and glomerules of the kidney are seen. Fatty changes, fibro blast proliferation and mitotic figures of the bileduct cells were observed.

E. Zearalenone

Pathology of Zearalenone in chicken include the presence of the oviduct and oestrogenic effects.

Histopathological examination showed cysts in the epithelium with chronic salphinigtis and peritonitis.

REFERENCES

Archilald, R.M., H.J. Smith and J.D. Smith, 1962. Brazilian groundnut toxidosis in Canandian broiler chickens. Can Vet J.3(1) : 322-325.

Asplin, F.D., and R.B.A. Carnaghan, 1961. The toxicity of certain groundnut meals for poultry with special reference to their effect on ducklings and chickens. Vet Rec. 73(3) : 1215-1219.

Bock, R.R.L., S. Shore, Y. Samberg and S. Perl. 1986. Death in broiler breeders due to salphingitis; possible role of Zearlenon. Avian Pathology 15(3) : 495-502.

Bodnarchuk, A.I., and IM., Kaspruk. 1984. Ochratoxicosis in Ducks. Poult. Abstr. 10 (5) : 1092 (Absrt).

Brown. T.P., R.O. Manning, O.J. Fletcher and R.D. Wyatt. 1986. The individual and combined effects of citrinin and ochnatoxin A on renal structure in layer chicks. Again diseases 30(1) : 191-198.

Burns, R.B. and. P. Dwivedi, 1986. The natural occurrence of ochratoxin A and its effects in poultry. A review II. Pathology and immunolgoy World Poultry Sci. 42(1) : 48-55.

Carlton, W.W, 1980. Citrinin : In conference on mycotoxins in Animal feed and grains related to animal health. pp. 275-323. Food and drug adm,. U.S. Dept of commerce. National Technical Information Service, USA.

Carnaghan, R.B.A., G. Lewis. D.S.P. Patterson and Ruth Allcroft 1966. Biochemical and pathological aspects of groundnut poisoning in chickens. Pathol. Vet 3 : 601-615.

Chang, C.F., J.A. Doerr and P.B. Hamilton, 1981. Comparitive study of T-2 toxin, orhratoxin and aflatoixn in broiler chicken. Poultry Sci. 60 (1) : 114-119.

Chang, C.F. and Hamilton, P.B. 1980. Ochratoxicosis in broiler chicken. Applied and environmental microbiology 39 (2) : 572-575.

Chang, C.F., W.E. Huff and P.B. Hamilton, 1979. A leucocytopenia induced in chickens by dietary ochratoxin. Poultry Sci. 58 (2) : 555-558.

Chi, M.S., C.J., Mirocha; Kurtz. H.J., G. A. Wearver, F. Bates, T. Robinson and Shimoda, W. 1980. Effect of dietary Zearalenone on growing broiler chicks, Poultry Sci. 59(3) : 531-536.

Dijkman, K.E., 1972. Aspergillus flavus infections in broiler and its significance in poultry carcas infection. Tijdischrift voor diergeness, Kunde, 97 : 1455.

Doerr, J.A., W. E. Huff and P.B. Hamilton, 1978. Enhanced Susceptiblity to bacterial toxins during aflatoxicosis. Poultry Sci. 57(4) : 1134.

Doupnik, B. and J.C., Peckham, 1970. Mycotoxicity of Aspergillus ochracens to chicks. Appl. microbiol 19 : 594-597.

Doerr, J.A., W.E. Huff and C.J. Wabeck. 1983. Effects of low level chronic aflatoxicosis in broiler chickens. Poultry Sci. 62 (10) : 1971-1977.

Dwivedi, P., and R.B. Burns, 1984. Pathology of chratoxicosis. A in young broiler chicks. Research in Vety. Science. 36 (1) : 92-103.

Dwivedi, P., and R.B., Burns, 1984. Effect of ochratoxin A on immunoglobulins in broiler chicks Research in Vet. Sci. 36 (1) : 117-121.

Dwivedi, P., R.B. Burns and M.H., Maxwell, 1984. Ultrastructural study of the liver and kidney in ochratoxicosis in young broiler chicks. Research in Vet. Sci. 36 (1) : 104-116.

Hamilton, P.B., W.E. Huff, Haris, Jr. U.R.D. Wyatt, 1982. Pathology of ochratoxin in broiler fowls. Poultry Sci. 16 (4) : 1832-1841.

Hinatov, L.L., and R.F. Wideman, Jr. 1985. Kidney function of single comb white leghorn pullets following acute renal portal poisoning of the mycotoxin. Citrinin. Poultry Sci. 64 (8) : 1553-1561.

Huff, W.E.R.D., Wyatt, T.L. Tucker and P.B.Hamilton, 1974. Ochratoxicosis in the broiler chickens. Poultry Sci. 53 (4) : 1585-1591

Huff, W.E., R.D. Wyatt, and P.B. Hamilton. 1975. Nephrotoxicity of Dietary ochratoxin A in Broiler chicken. Appl. miscrobial. 30 (1) 48-51.

Ivanovskii, A.A. 1986. Effect of sterigmato cystin on fowls and on the quality of poultry meat. Poultry Abstr. 12 (2) : 3085 (Abstr).

Mehdi, N.A.Q. W.W. Carlton and J. Tuite, 1981. Citrinin mycotoxicosis in broiler chickens. Food and Cosmetics Toxicology 19 (6) : 723-733.

Mehdi, N.A.Q. W.W. Carlton, G.D. Boon and J. Tuite, 1984. Studies on the sequentila development and pathogenesis of citrinin mycotoxicosis in turkeys and ducklings. Vet. Pathol. 21(2) : 216-223.

Meronuck, R.A., K. Garren, C.M. Christensen, G.H. Nelson and F. Bates, 1970. Effects on turkey poults and chicks of reations containing corn invarded by penillium and Fusarium species. Amen. J. Vet. Res. 31 (2): 551-555.

Moorthy, A.S., M. Mahender and P.R. Rao, 1985. Hepatopathology in experimental aflatoxicosi in chickens. Ind. J. of Anim. Sci. 55(2) : 629-632.

Muller, R.D., C.W. Carlson, G. Senenimick and G.S. Marshfiedl, 1970. The response of chicks, ducklings, gooslings, pheasants and poults to graded levels of aflatoxicosi. Poultry Sci. 49(4) : 1346-1350.

Peckham. J.C., B. Doupnik and O.H. Jones. 1971. Acute toxicity of ochnatoxins A and B in chicks. Appl. microbiol. 21 : 492-494.

Peckham, M. C. 1975. Poisons and Toxins. Diseases of Poultry Ed: Hofstad, M.S., B.W. Calnek, C.F. Elmboldt., W.W. Reid and H.W.Yadav, Jr. (1975). 6th edn., 1977. Oxford and IBH Publishing Co., India, pp 1134-1140.

Pohjanvirta, R.L. Sihvonen, and E. Karpanen, 1984. Suspected sterigmatocystin toxicosis in poultry. Vet. Bull. 54 (7) : 4241 (Abstr).

Speers, G.M., R. A. Meronuck, D.M. Barnes and C.J. Mirocha. 1971. Effects of feeding fusarium roseum F. sp. graminearum contamented corn and the cycotoxin F.2. on the growing chick and laying hen. Poultry Sci. 50(2) : 627-633.

Thaxton, P., H.T. Tung and P.B. Hamilton, 1974. Immunosupression in chickens by aflatoxin. Poultry Sci. 53 : 721.

Tung, H.T., J.W. Smith and P.B. Hamilton, 1971. Aflatoxicosis and bruising in the chicken. Poultry Sci. 50(3) : 795.

Threon, J.J., K.J. Vandermerwl, N. Liebenberg, H.J.B. Joubert, and W. Nle. 1986. Acute liver injury in ducklings and rate and a results of ochratoxin poisoning. J. Pathol. Bacterial. 91 (2) : 521-529.

Tucker, T, L., and P.B. Hamilton, 1971. The effect of ochratoxin in broilers. Poultry Sci. 50(5) : 1637 (Abstr.).

Tapia, M.O., J.A. Lopez and A.P. Casaro, 1980. Aflatoxocosis in broiler fowl. Poultry Abstr. 7 (7) : A. No. 1903.

Vanzytveld, W.A., D.C. Kelley and S.M. Dennis, 1970. Aflatoxicosis. The presence of aflatoxins or their metablities in livers and sekeletal muscles of chickens. Poultry Sci. 49 (4) : 1350-1356.

Wong, Z.A., and D.P.H. Hsieh, 1980. Comparative metabolism and toxicokinetics of aflatoxin B1 in the monkey, rat and mouse. Toxicol. Appl. Pharmacol. 55. 115.

Yadgiri, B. 1970. Aflatoxins toxicity in different sps of animals (cited from A.R. Reddy, M.V. Sci. theis. submitted to APAU, 1980.

Yoon, H.T. 1983. Studies on the toxicity of sterigmatocystin Korean Journal of Veterinary Public Health 7(2) : 85-91.

CHAPTER 34

MYCOTOXINS AND POULTRY HEALTH HAZARDS IN INDIA

Dr. S. M. Mohiuddin, Ph.D.
Associate Professor and Head Department of Pathology College of Veterinary Science Rajendranagar.

MAGNITUDE OF THE PROBLEM:

The increasing incidence of a number of unknown diseases in animals and poultry has been associated with ingestion of contaminated feed with biologically active compounds derived from the metabolic products of mould contaminants. It was only during 1961, the role of mycotoxins in the aetiology of disease in liverstock and poultry assumed considerable significance, after the outbreak of "Turkey" X disease resulting in heavy mortality when the birds were fed contaminated feed (Blount 1961). This appears to be possible in view of the ubiquituous distribution of the fungi and the favourable environmental conditions available in the tropical agroclimate for the growth during harvest and subsequent handling of crop.

It has been always noted that mould damaged feed ingridients which are unfit for human consumption, have been utilised in livestock and poultry feeds. The toxic symptoms arising from the consumption of moulds have recognised as mycotoxicosis.

FUNGAL CONTAMINATION:

Most species of the fungi associated with toxic diseases are saprophites and are widely distributed in nature. The tropical conditions in India, the harvesting practices and the post harvest storage practices with high temperature and high moisture during monsoon seasons, unseasonal rains and sudden flood grains provide favrourable conditions for the multiplication of the fungi and elaboration of mycotoxins.

Paddy cultivation is a major staple crop in many parts of India and in always harvested with high moisture constent, improper drying of paddy after parboiling process provides favourable immediately after harvesting contains high moisture winter seasons, provides favourable conditions for the production of higher levels of mycotoxins.

In Indian conditions the grains are stored (1) Under-ground. (2) Above ground and (3) root storage. These stored products exposed to rains leads to high moisture of the kernal of the food grains and the ubiquitous nature of the fungi leads to mouldy feeds. Certain insects also transmit spores of fungi, mostly. *A flavus* to grains, is evident from the work done at Central Food Technological Research Institute (Mysore). The commonly infesting fungi are *A flavus, A ochraceus* and *Pencilium* Islandicum (Srinath *et al.,* 1971, 1973). The most common contaminants recorded from the stored rice, sorgum and wheat is A. flavus (Rughunathan *et al.,* 1974).

FUNGAL INCIDENCE:

Oilseeds: Several studies were carried out to assess the incidence of fungal contamination in Indian conditions. The earliest studies carried out at the National Institute of Nutrition, found that 9% of the samples contained A. flavus and in 12% of the groundnuts samples Aflatoxin (Rao *et al.* 1965). The incidence of Aflatoxin in peanuts samples from Mysore state showed 150 isolates of *A. flavus,* Peanuts and groundnutt cake samples drawn from Gujarat state had higher level of higher level of toxin than from Andhra Pradesh and Madras (Sreenivasa Murthy *et al.,* 1965). Fairly high levels of Aflatoxin was found in 20-40% of kernels and 82% of oil cake (Anonymous, 1967). 50% of the 500 samples of groundnut from west coast contained Aflatoxin B, with a range of 0.10 to -.25 ppm (Wagle 1970). More than 50% of the 97 groundnut cake samples from Madhya Pradesh region contained Aflatoxin. Samples of 232 cotton seeds drawn from Maharashtra, Andhra and Gujarat contained Aflatoxin ranging from 50 ppb to 500 ppb (Raghavendra Rao *et al.,* 1970, Vadanayagam *et al.,* 1971)

CEREALS AND MILLETS:

In a study in the coastal district of Karnataka state *A. flavus, A candidus, Pencillium* citrninum were isolated from rice (Sreenivasa Murthy 1965) Screening of 300 samples of paddy, 70 samples of Jowar and 30 samples of ragi from the three regions of Andhra Pradesh revealed the presence of Alternaira, Dlechslera and curvularia. Also, screening for fungal contamination from rice, wheatmaize and pulses like tourdhal, Bengal gram and mung in and around Madras city contained, *Aspergillus, Penicilium, Alternaria, Furasarium, Heminthosporium Slachybotry* and *Pithomyces (Annonymous,* 1973). Curvularia Fusarium, Aspergillus and Penicilium species of fungus and Aflatoxins B_1, B_2, G_1, G_2 were noticed in sorgum grain in Pantnagar (Tripathy, 1973). Aflatoxin levels ranging from 5-15 ppm were recorded in maize grain and maize cobs from western Indian (Krishnan chari *et al.,* 1975b). Head moulds of Jowar from Hyderabad contained T2 toxin (Annonymous, 1976a). Investigation on the fungal contamination of poultry feed and mould food grains, revealed the presence of several toxigenic and non-toxigenic fungi (Kotch *et al.,* 1975, Jhala 1976).

It is evident from the available reports that there appears to be a predominance of *A. flavus* and occasionally *A. parasiticus* infection in India. Most of the isolates of *A. flavus* are toxigenic B_1, B_2 (Raghavendra Rao *et al.* 1970) and ludulkar *et al.,* 1971). Citrinin toxin was also isolated from groundnuts (Subramanyam and Rao 1974 b).

The following important diseases viz. (a) Aflatoxicosis, (b) Haemorrhagic syndrome (c) Nephropthy, caused by the consumption of mouldy feed in poultry are presented.

AFLATOXICOSIS:

There are several outbreaks of Aflatoxicosis in poultry in India, as could be seen from postmortem reports, but few were published. Heavy mortality due to Aflatoxicosis has been recorded in ducklings in the Government duck farm at Niranam, Kerala (Personal) communication) Raja Sekhara (1965) and Gopal (1986) studied the acute toxic effects in RIR chicks. An outbreaks of Aflatoxicosis causing from Karnataka (Gopal *et al.,* 1969). 50% mortality from the stock of 1000 birds was recorded by the authority in the Earn while you learn poultry Project at the College of Veterinary Science, Hyderabad in the year 1972. Death due to Aflatoxicosis was also reported in the tufted pochard ducks from Nehru Zoological Park. Hyderabad (Mohiuddin *et al.,* 1977).

The effect of the toxin may be either acute or chronic depending primarily on the dosage and frequency of exposure Secondly, it depends upon the age, sex, nutritional and physiological status. In majority of avain species studied death usually occurs within few days following acute toxicity and mild in chronic toxicity.

The first sign of the disease is in appearance and poor growth rate. Purple discoloration of comb, wattles, skin, shanks and lameness followed by ataxia, convulsors, opisthotonus and finally death.

Gross lesion in acute cases includes enlargement of liver, puffy, coloured kidneys were pale, slightly swollen petechial haemorrhages were noticed in liver, spleen, pancreas and in the intestine. In chronic cases the liver is shrunk, firm and hard and associated with ascitis.

The histological changes in acute cases were degenerative changes in hepatic cells of periportal zone in hepatic cells contain far globules in advanced cases, there will be karyohexis, karyolysis leading to death of the cell with mononuclear cell infiltration and over a cell proliferation. In chronic cases there is a variable degree of fatty change, bile ductular and masencymeral cell proliferation leading to bilary cirrhosis.

HAEMORRHAGIC SYNDROME:

Tripathy *et al.* (1967) recorded 22 deaths in a flock of R.I.R. pullets from Orissa. Variable degree of haemorrhages in subcutaneous tissues, muscles, liver, heart, spleen and kidneys were recorded (Sharma and Lingh, 1971). The disease was also recorded in Madras State (Damodaran, 1972). The author recorded 20-30% mortality of five outbreaks from Andhra Pradesh during 1971.

Although chemical, viral and bacterial agents have been studied as possible cause of the disease, the role of mycotoxins in the aetiology has not received adequate attention. The following fungi were reported to have a role in the aetiology via, Aspergillus, Pencillium and Altarnaria (Forgags and Carll 1955).

The lesions include subcutaneous and intra muscular haemorrhages, congestion of liver, fungus heart and gastro intestinal tract. Distorted focal necrotic areas, bile duct hyperplasia. Cholangtis, periduclutar fibrosis were observed, often with hyperptasia and hypertrophy of structular epithelum.

NEPHROPATHIC MYCOTOXIN (OCHRATOXIN):

Ochratoxin is a metabolite isolated from A ochratceous. It is first isolated from A ochraceous. If is first isolated and characterised by Vander. Mera *et al.* 1966. The toxin is subsequently reported from Pencilium viridictum, A mellaus A sulphureus (Lal *et al.*, 1968 and 1970). The toxin is represented by three similar compounds to which ochratoxin, A. (2H 18oC Ncl) is mostly toxic and abundant. The moulds are widely distributed in soil and decaying organic matter and frequently associated with mouldy feed (Shot Well *et al.*, 1968, 1969).

In chicks delayed sexual maturity, lowered egg production reduced hatchability and depressed further performance of the progeny was reported (Chowdhury *et al.*,1971). Hepatic lesion were less frequent than renal. The changes in kidneys are characterised by degeneration of proximal tubules interstitial fibrosis and development of sclerotized glomerula tuff (Krogh, 1975). The hepatic lesion vary in saverity from mild diffuse vacuolation to necroitc foci (Chowdhary *et al.*, 1971). Naphropathic of Mycotoxins has not been recorded in India.

SUMMARY

In this paper an attempt has been made to highlight the magnitude of the problem. "Mycotoxins and Health Hazards in poultry in India". The incidence of fungal contamination of different crops, oilseeds, cereals and millets with different species of fungi and the levels of the toxins present in those grains were also presented. The following important diseases (a) Aflatoxicosis, (b) Haemor tragic syndrome, (c) Nephropathy mycotoxin in the poultry were presented in detail.

REFERENCES

Annonymous (1966), Annual report 1966-67, Regional Research, Laboratory, Hyderabad.

Annoymous (1973). Report of FL-480 protect UR No. A (10)- 97, University Biochemical Laboratories, Madras.

Annonymous (1076a), Annual report N.N. Hyderabad.

Blount, W.P. (1961). J. Brit, Turkey, Fed: 9-52.

Damodaran S (1978). Seminar on Avian Diseases, IVRI.

Forgag's Carbl. W.T. (1055). Vet. Ved. 50-172.

Gopal, T. (1966), M.V.Sc. Dissertation, University of Madras.

Gopal. T. and Zuki, Narayannaswamy, M. and Prelata S. (1969). Ind. Vet. Jour. 46 : 348.

Indulkar, A.S. Vedanayagam S and Rao S.R. (1971, Second international Symposium on plant pathology, IAR, New Delhi.

Jhala, V.M. (1936), Ind. Vet. Jour. 53-401.

Kotch, R.E., Bhiwmick K.B.D. and Kotch B.S. (1975). Ind, Vet. Jour. 52-759.

Koragh, P. (1975), Inst. Nation, diseases Animal, Vol. 46-57.

LaimMc, E., Semeuk G. and Hessletine G.M. (1968). Phytopathology, 88-1050.

Krishnamachari K.A.V.R., Bhat R.V., Nagaraian V. and Tilak T.B. (1975b), Ind; Jour. Med. Res. 63-1036.

Lai, M.CE., Semenuk, G. and Hessaletine C.M. (1970), Appl, Microbiol, 19-542.

Mohiuddin, S.M. and Gowher Ali Md. (1977). Ind. Vet. Jour. 54-84.

Rajesekharan. D. (T965). M.V.Sc. Dessertation, University of Madras.

Rao, K.S., Madhavan, T.V. and Tulpule P.S. (1965), Ind. Jour. Med. Res. 53-1196.

Raghavendra Rao, S., Indulkar A.S. and Vedanayagam, H.S. (1970), Report of PL 480 project No. A7 MQ-17, Regional Research, Laboratory, Hyd.

Raghunathan, A.N., Srinath, D. and Majumdev, S.K. (1974), J. Food Sic. Technol.

Sreenivasamurthy, V., Jayaraman, A. and Parpia H.A.B. (1-65). Aflatoxin in Indian Peanuts (G.N. Wagan ed) PP 251, M.I.T. Press, Cambridge, Mass.

Srinath, D., Raghunathan, A.N. and Mujumdar, S.E. (1971), Second Int. Symp Plant, Pathol, New Delhi, P. 32.

Sharma, W.K. and Lingh, N. (1971), Ind. Vet. Journ.

Sirnath, D. Raghunathan, A.N. and Majumdar S.K. (1973), Curr. Sci. 42-683.

Subrahmanyam, P. and Rao, A.S. (1974b). Unvi. Sci. 43-707.

Tripathy, S.B., Nayak, N.C. and Mohanty K.M. (1967) Ind. Vet. Jour 44-813

Tripathi, R.K. (1973), Ind, Jour, Exp. Biol. 11: 361.

Vedanayagam, H.S. Indulkar A.S. and Rao S.R. (1971), Ind, Jour, Exp. Biol. 9 : 410.

Wag E.N.G. (1970), Indian Stand Ind Bull 22 : 299.

CHAPTER

35

MYCOTOXICOSIS AND ITS CONTROL

Dr. S.M. Mohiuddin
Protener Professor & Head Department of Pathology C.V.Sc., R'nagar, Hyd. 0-30

Mycotoxine are defined as fungi-metabolites produced in feed stuffs which can cause disease and death in man and animals. There is now a growing awareness of the implication of mycotoxin as frequent contaminants of agricultural commodites and their associated health and economic hazzards.

There are over 200 fungai known to produce the mycotoxins we know little about the toxicity of a few of these toxins. The important mycotoxine identified are aflatoxins, ochratoxisn, trichothecense, citrinin and Zearlaenone. These toxic agents are ubiquitous in distribution and have been isolated from a wide variety of food and mixed feeds.

Contamination of feed:

About 100 fungi that grow on standing cross or stored feeds are known to produce toxic substance and about 20 of these substances have been associated with naturally-occuring diseases in man and animals.

In majority of the cases the fungal contamination occurs during harvesting. Improper storage of feed ingredients and mixed feeds become contaminated with fungi. Many fungi are oppotunistic pathogens which can invade and produce mycotoxins when the grain is in the field.

A moisture content of 12% and above in the feed relative humidity of 80-90% and temperature ranging from 10°C to 42°C is sufficient for prolific fungal growth. All these conditions are available in tropical countries like India.

Many of the mycotoxins are hear-stable and survive palleting, canning and other processing-operations. Mycotoxins, are also nonantigenic. Except aflatoxins, very little information is available regarding pathogenesis, or clinical effects of acute and chronic affects of these toxins and diagnosis.

Effects of mycotoxins

Among the various mycotoxins, aflatoxins are considered to be the most potent and harmful. Aflatoxin are the metabolic products of the fungi *Aspergillus flavus* and *Aspergillus Parasiticus.* They produce aflatoxins B1, B2, G1, G2 M1 and M2. Among these aflatoxin B1 is highly toxic and harmful.

Aflatoxins are primarily hepatotoxic, secondarly Carcinogenic, Teratogenic and Mustogenic. Its effects on poultry production are:

1) Reduce bodyweight gain.
2) Decrease egg production as well as egg weight.
3) Suppresses the immune-system, making them highly susceptible to diseases.
4) Disrupts bone development causing ricketic type problems.
5) Induce many nutritional problems through its effects on nutrient absorption and metabolism.
6) Causes bruises in broilers resulting in condemnation of the carcass.
7) Lower hatchability and increase embryonic mortality.
8) Economic effects of Mycotoxins and Aflatoxins on poultry reduced rate of Egg production.

Dose	Egg production	Egg weights
(PPM)	%	(gm)
0.00	81.7	56.7
1.25	74.6	57.2
2.50	85.2	55.2
5.00	72.2	55.6
10.00	26.8	51.3

In another study at National Institute of Nutrition, Hyderabad it was found that feeding of 0.7 ppm of aflatoxins contaminated feed for a short duration had resulted in over 30% reduction in egg production and loss of over Rs. 45,000/- over a three-weeks-period occurred in a farm with 11,000 layers.

Another mycotoxin, Ochratoxin, is primarily a hephrotoxin in poultry. Ochratoxin is three times more toxic than aflatoxin to broiler chickens. T2 toxins is a diemetric toxin and its action is similar to radiation.

Mycotoxins interactions:

Several analytical laboratories have found that most mycotoxin contaminated samples contain more than just a single mycotoxin. When aflatoxin and Ochratoxin are co-contaminants of poultry feed they interact in synergistic manner, i.e. the toxicity that results from dual exposure to aflatoxin and Ochratoxin is more severe than the sum of the individual toxicity of these mycotoxins. This may be one reason why very low levels of aflatoxin in the field could produce significant ill affects in poultry compared to laboratory studies Where only a single mycotoxin is studied. Due to interaction the symptoms are also different. The target organ of the interaction between aflatoxin and though the interaction is antagonist, the animals perform such more poorly in the interaction group when compared to growing animals on just a single toxin. The mycotoxin combinationof aflatoxin and T-2 toxin is found to exhibit a synergistic affect.

Mycotoxin safe limits:

Opinion is unanimous as far as the affects of aflatoxin on poultry production are concerned. However, as far as the tolerable level of aflatoxin is concerned there is total diversity of opinion. Levels ranging from 20 ppb to 2000 ppb have been founded about as "safe" level. One of the reasons for such wide-ranging claim is that may studies have taken mortality as a criterion for defining safe limits. However in poultry farming it is not enough to just keep the birds alive without production, which matters more.

The European Economic Community (EEC) limit of 20 ppb (incorporated into the legislation of all member states) assumed significance. While it may be argued that this limit is not totally applicable to Indian conditions, what is signifcant is that this limit was fixed, keeping in view two well defined parameters, namely that the allowed levels for aflatoxin should not.

1) Impair the health of animals and hence it is productive.
2) Be sufficient to enter the human food chain via animal products.

To determine the relative safety of a feed based one single

mycotoxin analysis may grossly underestimate the true risk we are taking. Many factors are found to effect the toxicity of aflatoxin and these include (a) genetic variability (b) nutritional status of the animal (c) environmental stress, and (d) sex differences. Thus safety is a concept that is usually based on the individuals limited experience, even very minute doses over a prolonged period may prove to be carcinogenic.

Aflatoxn levels: Data on Aflatoxin levels analysed in different feed ingredients, from June 1988 to March 1990.

S. No.	Samples	No. of samples analysed	Aflatoxin +ve	Percentage of incidence	Toxin levels ppm.
1.	Compound feed	211	102		0.02-0.4
2.	C.N. cake	169	94		0.01-0.8
3.	Fish	32	10		0.01-0.2
4.	Maize	41	11		0.01-0.4
5.	Liver Meal	9	9		0.01-0.8
6.	Meat Meal	2	2		0.4
7.	Bajra	7	3		0.1-0.2
8.	Soya Bean meal	5	4		0.1-0.2
9.	Till cake	2	2		Below 0.05
10.	Sunflower cake	2	2		0.01-0.2

Methods of prevent mycotoxicosis:

Mycotoxicosis is a global problem which is very difficult to tackle. The control methods tried include the following:

1. Establishing a mycotoxn-screening program.
2. Careful monitoring and controlling of the moisture level of feed ingredient.

3. Periodically cleaning all feed handling equipment with a 5% to 210% bleaching solution.
4. Keeping the time from manufacture of feeds to presentation to the animals at a a minimum.
5.. Minimising pellet breakdown to reduce the level of fineness in the feed.
6. Using a mould inhibitory to prevent further contamination of feed ingredients and mixed feeds and
7. Using feed-additives to reduce the toxicity of aflatoxin.
8. Detoxification inactivation of mycotoxin contaminated food and feed have been proposed.

They are (a) the ammoniation of the grains and feed stuffs told destroy aflatoxin and (b) the addition of "sorbet" to the grains and feed stuff destroy the aflatoxin.

In conclusion, mycotoxins have been recognised as significant economic and health hazzards on worldwide scale. A concerned interdisciplinary research effort involving the academic, Government and Industrial agencies to develop viable measures to solve this important problems is clearly warranted at this juncture.

CHAPTER 36

EFFECTS OF AFLATOXIN ON IMMUNE RESPONSE IN VIRAL DISEASE

S.M. Mohiuddin
College of Veterinary Science, Rajendranagar, Hyderabad

INTRODUCTION

It is assumed that Aflatoxins have greater importance than other mycotoxins, since apart from their hepatotoxic, effects they are immuno-suppressive. It is well known that mouldy damaged feed ingredients which are unfit for human consumption have been utilised in livestock and poultry feed.

MATERIAL AND METHODS

Humoral and cell-mediate imune response was studied in birds fed with Aflatoxin orally 100 mg/chick and 200 mg/ chick for 21 days from the 4th week onwards to group II and III respectively, while group III and IV were fed with vit A 1000 IU/birds/day respectively. Group I birds were maintained on toxin free diet. Blood samples were collected for haematological and serum samples for antibody after 14 days from groups I-V, All the chicks, were vaccinated with Ranikhet disease (R2B strains) vaccine. Again on the 7th day post-vaccination booster dose of RD (R2B strains) vaccine was given. All the chickens were maintained on their respective diet for another 7 days, blood samples and serum were collected for analysis from all the groups.

Tissue phagocytic activity was studied in five cockrels, fed with Aflatoxin mixed feed at 20 ppm while the control (two cockrels) were maintained on toxin-free diet for three months. Then 1 ml of saturated carbon solution was injected i/v through wing vein. All the birds were sacrificed after 48 hours live collected to study the cells phagocytic actively through histological parameters.

In the third experiment thirty boiler chicken of 5 weeks age were divided into three groups having ten birds in each group. Group II and III were fed with 1.0 ppm and 2.5 ppm of Aflatoxin prepared from *Aspergillus parasiticus* culture in rice, mixed in feed respectively.

While group I maintained on toxin-free diet for a period of three weeks. Alpha Naphthyl Estrase (ANAE) activity in blood smears and separated phagocytes was studied and Adenosine Deaminase Estrases (ADE) activity was studied in blood smears and serum.

RESULTS AND DISCUSSION

I. Studies on the effects off Aflatoxin on antibody synthesis against Ranikhet Disease (RD) vaccine in chicks.

In this study it has been concluded that feeding of aflatoxin @ 100 mg daily/chick for 14 days, prior to vaccination did not affect the haematological total count and differentia count studies. The effect of feeding 100 mg and 200 mg of Afltoxin daily for 14 days before R.D. vaccination was similar, but further feeding of Aflatoxin @ 200 kg for 21 days after RD, vaccination resulted in increased serum-Alkaline phosphatase activity, increase RBCs fragility and decease in antibodies without any change in other parameters studied. Administration of Vit. A gave protection against. Aflatoxin, but failed to enhance the immunity. Thus feeding of Aflatoxin 0.1 do poultry during stress of vaccination did not interfere with any biochemical activities whereas feeding with 0.2 ppm interfere with biochemical changes and immunity production. Thus is concluded that humoral immunity is affected at feeding 0.2 ppm to 4 weeks old chicks for a period of 1 days after vacciantion.

II Studies on phagocytic activity and haematological changes in Aflatoxicosis in Poultry.

In this study it is concluded that the birds for aflatoxin at 200 ppm over a period of three months showed a decrease in phagocytic activity of heterophils, kuffer cells and haemotological values. The total Basophilic and Thromobocytic counts were decreased, suggesting that Aflatoxins lowers the resistance of the body leading to increase in the incidence of infectious diseases. The study suggest that cell mediated immune response is affected.

III. Enumaration of T. lympchocytes and Adenosine Deaminase Estrases activity in lymphodcytes and serum in Aflatoxin-fed birds.

In this study thirty broiler chicks were reared upto four weeks of age and they were divided into from three groups. Group I served as control and was fed with Aflatoxin at 1.0 ppm and 2.5 ppm respective for three weeks. All these birds were sacrificed, blood smears. lymphocytes from peripheral bloodand serum were collected for analysis.

Quantiatiative estimation of T. lymphocytes in the blood smear was carried out using Alpha Naphthiyl Acetate Estrase (ANAE) staining method which give one or two reddish brown reaction productions in the The ANAE positive cell count (T. lymphocytes) in the blood in control group is 36.0 ± 4.34 while in group II is 26.0 ± 1.50 and in group III is 24.1 ± 1.22. There is a statistically significant decrease ($p<0.01$) in T. lymphocytes in group II and III.

Alpha Naphthly Acetate Estrase (ANAE) staining has been shown to be a reliable cytochemical marks for identification of Monoecytes and T. lymphocytes in peripheral blood (Muller *et al.,* 1979). Aflalatoxin feeding in the two groups resulted in a significant decrease of T. lymphocytes thus affecting the cell mediated immune response. This confirms the lymphopenia noticed in aflatoxicosis by Campbell and Deorr, (1981).

Adenosine Deaminase Estrases (ADE) is separate lymphocytes and serum.

The DNA is one of the enzymes of purine salvage pathway. Of late the role of purine metabolismin the immune response has gained importance.

The need of proliferating cells for a balanced supply of both purine and pyramidien compounds for maintaining cell division and growth has long been known. But the importance of pathways of purine inter-conversion in maintaining the integrity of the striking has been revealed by the striking impairment of its function found in association with deficiencies of specific enzyeme of purine metablolism. The first enzyme defect to be found in association with severe immunodeficiency disease in ADE (Giblet *et al.,* 1972). The lymphocytic ADE could severe as a marker of cell mediated immunity.

The lymphocyte ADE activity in group I was 50.28 ±9.5 group II 49.25± 18.24 and group III 20.78. 10.5 nanomoles of amrad a liberated/ million cells/hour. There was a significant decrease ($P<0.01$) in the lympocytic ADE in group II and III hence convincingly be concluded that the inhabitation of proliferation of T-cell is by Aflatoxins.

The serum ADE activity did not show any significant differences amongst the groups I, II and III. The activity in group I is 6.60±2.04, group II 5.64=2.05 and group III is 4.84 ±1.65 1.U/ml serum.

REFERENCES

Campbell, J.M.L. and Doerr, J.A. (1981), *Poul. Sci.,* **60** : 1633.

Giblett, E.R. Anderson, J.E., Cohen F., Pollara, B. and Mezwissen, H.J. (1972), *Lancet* , **2** : 1067.

Mueller, J. Burn De. Re. G., Bucki A., Keller, H.U. and Cottier, H., (1979), *European, J. Immul.,* **5** : 270.

CHAPTER 37

HANDLING MYCOTOXIN CONTAMINATED FEEDSTUFF

Dr. S.M. Mohiuddin

During recent years, voluminous information has been accumulated on mycotoxin production, mechanism, of action and their effects in livestock and poultry. The need of the hour is to know how to utilise mycotoxin contaminated feed in livesstock poultry rations.

Since the outbreak of Turkey X-disease in Britain during 1960 worldwide attention has been directed at a thorough investigation of mycotoxicisis. There are more than 300 fungi known to produce mycotoxins but we know little about the toxocity they produce excepting a few toxins. The important mycotoxins identified are aflatoxins, ochratoxins, trichothecene, citrinin and zearzloenone. These toxic agents are ubiquitous in distribution and have been isolated from a wide variety of grains and mixed feeds.

Aflatoxin

Among the various mycotoxins, aflatoxins are considered to be the most potent and harmful for they are hepatotoxic, mutagenic carcinogenic, antimytotic and immunosuppressive in their effects and no other toxin has such a wide range of activity and hence it has created great awareness throughout the world. Aflatoxins are the products of fungi, aspergillus, flavus and aspergilus parasiticus. They produce aflatoxins B1, B2, G2, M1, M2. Among these the most harmful and most is B1.

Fungal Growth

Aspergillus belongs to the family Aspergillaecae. In a majority of cases the fungal contamination occurs during harvesting transport, improper storage of feed ingredients and mixed feed. a moisture content of 12% of and above in the feed and relative humidity of 80-90% and temperature ranging between 10-42°C is sufficient for prolific growth of fungi.

Many of the mycotoxins are heat stable and survive pelleting and other processing operations. Many mycotoxins are non-antigenic. Excepting aflatoxins, little information is available regarding pathogenesis, clinical acute and chronic toxic effects and diagnosis of these toxins.

Mycotoxin safe limits

As far as the toxic effects of aflatoxin is concerned there is a total diversity of opinion. Levels ranging from 20 ppb to 2000 ppb have been suggested as "safe levels'. One of the reasons for such a wide ranging claim is that many studies have taken only mortality as the criteria for defining safe limits. However if poultry farming it is not enough just to keep the birds alive without prodction, which matters.

The European Economic Community (EEC) of limit of 20 ppb (incorporated into the legislation of significance. This limit was fixed keeping in view two well defined parameters. That allowed level of aflatoxin should not: i) impair the health of animals and its productivity. ii) to be sufficient to enter the human food chain via animal products.

To determine the selective safety of feed based on single mycotoxin analysis may grossly underestimate the true risk. Many factors are found to affect the toxicity of aflatoxin, these include genetic, variability, nutritional status of the animal, environmental stress, age and sex differences.

Thus, the safety in a concept that is usually based on the individual's limited experience. It has been stressed that there can be no safe level of mycotoxins, as even minute doses over a pro longed period may prove to be carcinogenic.

Effects on Aflatoxin

Mycotoxins causes a wide variety of clinical signs in poultry and livestock. They are primarily hapatoxic, but affect all the systems in the individual, leading to gross and hisotpathological changes affecting growth and productivity and finally leading to increased mortality. Besides, aflatoxins are mutagenic, carcinogenic, and antimytotic in activity. They also affect immunological system and hence the birds are also susceptible to many infectious and conagious diseases. In chronic conditions explicit clinical signs are absent except for a slight reduction in productivity and hence often it remains unidentified.

Aflatoxin levels analysed in different ingredients in Andhra Pradesh, India.

Sl. No.	Samples	Samples Analysed	Aflatoxin present	Toxin levels ppm
1	Compound feed	211	102	0.002-0.4
2.	Ground Nut cake	169	94	0.01-0.3
3.	Fish	32	10	0.01-0.2
4.	Maize	41	11	0.01-0.4
5.	Liver meal	9	9	0.01-0.3
6.	Meat meal	2	2	0.4
7.	Bajra	7	3	0.10-0.2
8.	Soyabean meal	5	4	0.10-0.2
9.	Til cake	2	2	Below 0.05
10.	Sunflower cake	2	2	0.10-0.2

Decontamination Techniques

It is estimated that mycotoxin affects as much as 40% of the world food crops each year. Mycotoxicosis occurred naturally in wide variety of crops used as foodstuff, which support the growth of fungi. Crops that contain toxin-producing fungi may not yet be contaminated with mycotoxins. However, the mere presence of the toxin-producing strain, indicates a potential hazard. Also individual moulds or mycotoxins rarely occur in isolation. Two or more mycotoxins together may have a greater toxic effect than on any individual basis. Killing these organisms may stop the production of toxin but does not remove the mycotoxins already present in the feed. Hence the biggest challenges in coping with mycotoxin contaminated feed-stuffs is to identify the types of toxins and concentrations quickly. The principle method adopted for preventingmycotoxicosis is preventive treatment using feed additives and enzymes.

Preventive Treatment

The first effort to decontaminate the contaminated feed grains is through liquid extraction using organic solvents or water-based solution of calcium chloride or sodium bicarbonate or by heated salt water. Ammonia treatment and treatment with monomethylamine and calcium lydroxide may also be effective. Toxins can also be destroyed of heat and pressure in the presence of heat and pressure in the presence of moisture. However the utility of this treatment depends upon the type of mycotoxin, heating time; the temperature and water content of the feed grains. Some mycotoxins such as water-free aflatoxins, trichothecene, zeralenone, chloratoxin, patulin and pencillic acid are highly stable, whereas ergot alkaloids and citrinin, which usually occur in grains like wheat and rye, are easily destroyed by heat. Ultraviolet (UV) ray and ionising radiation is also effective in destroying some mycotoxins such as aflatoxins, but it also destroys the nutrient in the feed stuffs. However, the ammonia detoxification of aflatoxin is the most practical, widely adopted and most useful method.

Using Feed additives

The practical difficulties encountered in preventative treatment of contaminated feeds, the cost involvement and the time-consuming process have focused the need to use feed additives in the rations. These feed additives may be incorporated into the feed products to become active in vivo against mycotoxins.

Some mineral compounds are capable of absorbing or trapping mycotoxin molecules and isolate the molecules from being absorbed and digested without harmful to the animals. These compounds are commonly referred as feed additives, such as, activated charcoal, yeast cell wall product and mined mineral clays like sodium bentonites and sepiolites havethis capacity to a varying degree.

The synthetic products used are zeolite, alumino silicate and gamma amino butric acid (GABA). Zeolite is effective against aflatoxin, T-2 toxin or vomitoxin, but the compound is not specific and usually binds, incompletely with number of toxins.Adding zeolite at 2% level of the aflatoxin B-1 1 mg/kg contaminated feed its reduced concentration in the liver to 30-40%. The addition of 0.02% of DL methionine to be mixed feed drastically reduces the effect of zeolite. There is also a possibility of medicines reducing the efficiency of mycotoxin binding capacity.

The toxins in the feed after absorption reach the liver for detoxification and first of all, it reduces the efficiency of energy exchange. As the heat production in poultry increases the energy deficit of endogenic nature appears, which leads to a reduction of positive feed energy (PFE). The addition of such substances to feed, which normalises the energy exchange, makes it possible to weaken the action of mycotoxins if concentration if high or prevent the reduction of productivity if there is only low toxin consumption Gamma amino butyric acid (GABA) and its analogue, as well as succinic acid were tested as substances which normalise the energy exchange.

The addition of gamma amino butyric acid (GABA) to feed containing 1 mg/kg feed aflatoxin, is highly effective against the toxic effects and when the toxin level is 2mg/kg feed but its effect is not total.

Alumino-silicate added to the contaminated feed has the effective absorbing capacity to aflotoxin, and to a limited extent to zerolenone and B trichothrcene.

Methionine Supplementation

Mycotoxins are absorbed by blood and are detoxified in the liver. In detoxifying aflatoxin in the liver by biological reduction, oxidation reaction is based upon glutathione. Glutathione is partly composed of methionines and cystine. Therefore there is depletion of methionine which will affect growth and performance. Hence it is also recommended that in addition of extra quantity of methionine when aflatoxin contaminated based feed is fed.

Uses of enzymes

The newest technique developed for decontamination of mycotoxin involves the help of enzymes to decompose the toxin. With the knowledge and understanding that most of the mycotoxins are subjected to the mycotoxins are subjected to bio-transformation by microsonal oxidise of liver, the thought is to made use of each substances which enhances enzymatic activity in the metabolism of mycotoxins (mono-oxygenases inductors (MO)). The enzymes degrade a toxin by breaking the molecules apart to form hairless metabolies. The metabolies thus created are less toxic can easily and quickly be removed from the organism, resulting in the reduction of the toxin concentration in the liver and thus decreasing the toxic influences. Enzymes are availed to inactivate zearalenone, t-2 toxin, deoxynivalenol, nirolenol and diacetoxyscirpenal. The enzyme estrase, breaks the lactone ring of zearalenone, while the enzyme epoxidase degrades the 12, 13 epoxy group in the trichothecens. By breaking apart the functional atomic groups within the mycotoxin molecules the enzymes renders them non-toxic. As non-toxic metabolites, the degraded mycotoxin are digested or excreted without causing any harmful effects.

In conclusion, what is unwanted for human consumption cannot be thrown out. This has to be reutlised in livestock and poultry rations. The management of the risk of mycotoxin contaminated feed in the rations is the most important aspect of the recent approaches to the problem.

There are a number of techniques used to lower the risk of toxicity:

- Establishing a mycotoxin screening programme.
- The first line of defence is preventing mould infestation and mycotoxin in the field. The grains need to be harvested, dried and stored properly to prevent conditions leading to mycotoxin production during storage.
- The basic common sense approach is to segregate physically damaged or fungi infested kernels or seeds.
- If possible, reduce the impact by modifying animal diets, diluting toxic grains with clean grains and improving the nutritional content of the diet.
- Adding mould inhibitors to prevent further contamination of feeds.
- Using feed additives to reduce toxicity of feed.
- A recent approach is to use enzymes.
- Methionine supplementation so about 30-340% over NRC recommendations reduces toxic effects.

CHAPTER

38

AN OVERVIEW OF MYCOTOXICOSIS

Prof. S.M. Mohiuddin,
Rtd. Professor of Pathology, Gaffar Khan Colony, Road No. 10,
Plot No. 76 Banjara Hills Hyderabad - 34 A.P.

For the past 38 years considerable progress has been made in the study of Mycotoxins and improving the methods of analyses, yet there are many problems.

By some, it is estimated that Mycotoxin affects as much as 40% of the world food crops every year. Most Mycotoxins are chemically stable and persist long after the Mycotoxins-producing fungi are destroyed.

Because most commercial Poultry Producers, especially Broiler producers feed grains and oil seed based diet wherein Mycotoxins represents a significant, continuing risk to profitability.

Mycotoxins occur naturally in a wide variety of crops used in fed stuffs that support the growth of the fungi are:

Crop	Mycotoxins contamination
1. Alfalfa/lucern	Aflatoxin, Zearalenone.
2. Barley	Aflatoxin, Don, Niv, T-2 toxin, DAS, Zearalenone, Ochratoxin-A, Streigmatocysin, Citrinin, Viomellein, Zanthomegnin, Vioxanthin.
3. Cassava/topioca	Aflatoxin, Zearlenone.
4. Cotton seed	Aflatoxin
5. Ground nuts/peanuts	Aflatoxin, Cyclopiazonic acid, ochratoxin-A, Citrinin, Zearalenone, Verruculotoxin,

6. Maize/com	Aflatoxin, Zearalenone, DOD, T-2, DAS, Niv. Butenolide, moniliformis, Furmoniliformin, fumonisin, Secatonic acid
7. Maize Silage	Patlin
8. Oats	Aflatoxin, DON, T-2 toxin, NS, HT-2, Zearalenone, Ochratoxin-A, Citrinin.
9. Rye	Aflatoxin, DON, NIV, Zearalenone, Ochratoxin-A, Citrinin, Ergotalkaoids.
10. Rice	Aflatoxin, Zearalenone, Ochratoxin-A, Sterigmatocystin, Citrinin.
11. Ryegrass	Egrotalkaloids, Sporidesmins, Lolitrems
12. Sorgum/Milo	Afltoxins, T-2, Toxins, Zearalenone, Ochratoxin-A
13. Soyabean/Soya	Aflatoxins
14. Wheat	Citrinin, Ergotalkaloids, Viomellin, Znathomegnin, Vioxanthin.
15. Wheat Straw	Salratoxins, Roridins.
DON : Deoxynivalenol	NIV : Nivabenol
DAS : Diacetoxyscirpenol	NS : Neosalanoil

Also individual moulds fungi or Mycotoxins rarely occur alone or in isolation. Two or more Mycotoxins together may have a greater toxic effect than any one on individual basis.

A special consideration for feed manufactures is that milling by products such as Bran, middling and "mill run" materials may contain higher concentrations of Mycotoxins than refined meal or flour. This is because fungal infestation is first likely to concentrate in broken or damaged kernels or seeds in which the seed coat or longer protects the starchy interior. However, such milling byproducts especially from wheat four production are less rigorously delaminated for Mycotoxins than are whole grains.

One of the biggest challenges in coping with Mycotoxins in feed stuff is to identify types and concentrations quickly in the field prior to harvest, immediately post-harvest, at the grain terminal or the feed mills.

Toxins Estimation

The various methods known for estimation are

1. Thin layer Chromatography (T.L.C.):

This method suffers from insensitivity, it only decides the presence of Mycotoxins.

2. HPLC Method

More accurate, individual toxin can be separated.

3. Immunosassy:

Mostly Elisas (enzyme Linked Immuno absorbent Assey).

This method is applied as a rapid method for screening and monitor the presence or absence of a particular Mycotoxins. The main drawback of Elisa still often is only the semiquantitative nature of the results.

European economic community (E.E.C.) limit:

E.E.C was introduced by 1976, set criteria that the allowed levels for aflatoxin should not:

a. Impair the health of animal and its productivity.

b. Be not sufficient to enter the human food chain via animal products.

In a study conducted by Prof. S. Mohiuddin, "Feeding trails on aflatoxin", showed presence of 200 mg/day for 14 days prior to vaccination with R.D. Further feeding of aflatxin for 21 days results in decreased SAD activity and R.B.C.S. fragility and decreased antibody titres as against feeding 100 mg/bird/day. Thus, it is concluded feed of aflatoxin at 0.2 PPM fed to 4 weeks old chicks for a period of 21 days affected antibody titres.

In another study Prof. Mohiuddin concluded that feeding of 200 PPM aflatoxin over a period of 3 months showed decreased phagocytic

Hissar Agricultural (University Levels)	CARI levels
These limits are based on foreign literature and have no relevance under Indian conditions. This is because the standards of performance is much superior in western countries than in India.	Indian reference are few but show remarkably different findings.
300 PPb in Poultry	White Leghorn
300 PPb in Pigs	Chicks 150 PPb
600 PPb in Cattle	Pure breed broiler chickes 200 PPb
1750 PPb in sheep	Cross breed broiler chicken 400 PPb
	Quil starter chickens 300 Pb
	Guinea Foul Kitls - 150 PPb

Sl. No.	Added of the main ration	Live weight at 7 weeks age (g)	Feed of consumption/1kg of weight gian (kg)	Aflatoxin content in the liver (mg/kg)
1.	-	1981±43	2.00	0.00
2.	2 mg/kg. Aflatoxin	1542±43	2.85	187±1.6
3.	2 mg/kg Aflatoxin + Zeolite	1728±4.30	2.26	147±0.9
4.	2 mg/kg Aflatoxin + Gaba	1624±28	2.43	16.2±1.6
5.	2 mg/kg Aflatoxin + Zelogram	1848±51(.)	2.17	1.34±(X)

activity of heterophills, kuffer cells, and haematological value, which suggest that cell mediated immuno response is affected.

Toxicity:

The toxicity may be acute or chronic. The problems of diagnosis is acute toxicity is easier than chronic, because the symptoms in acute are prominent and definite.

Whereas, in chronmic toxicity, the symptom appear a week or two after feeding after toxic feed and the symptoms are only a slight reduction in production, which might be due to many other causes. Hence, such toxicity remain unidentified over a longer time. There is also a number of difficulties related to be a intricacy of identifying such chronic Mycotoxicity.

Decontaminant techniques:

Early efforts to decontaminate Mycotoxin contaminated grains invoved.

i. Liquid extraction: Using organic solvents or water base solutions of calcium chloride or sodium bicarbonate:

A degree of decontamination can be achieved by extraction with heated salt water. This is relatively economic and causes fewer problems in animal health; but, requires considerable handling time, equipment and labour.

ii. Ammonia treatment, and treatment with monomethylamine and Calcium Hydroxide:

May be effective under proper controlled conditions.

iii. It is also possible to destroy most Mycotoxins with heat or a combination of heat and pressure especially in the presence of moisture:

However, sensitivity to heat depends upon the type of mycotoxin, heaitng time and temperature and the water content of the feed stuff.

Some Mycotoxins, such as water-free Aflatoxins, Trichothecene toxins (such as deoxynivalenol) Zearalenone. Ochratoxin-A, Patulin and Panicillic acid are highly stable:

By contrast egotalkaloids and citrinin-which usually occur in the temperature fine grains such as wheat and rage-are relatively easy to destroy by heating.

iv. Ultraviolet and lonising radiation:

May be effective in destroying some Mycotoxins, such as Aflatoxins, but are likely to destroy nutrient also in the feed stuff. Thus, for practical and commercial detoxification of Mycotoxin only Ammoniation is able to destroy Aflatoxin.

Feed Additives (Toxin Binders):

Some mineral compounds are capable of absorbing or traping Mycotoxin molecules. "Adsorption" refers to attachment of Mycotoxins molecules to the surface of other harmless molecules and is different from"Absorption". Adsorption isolates the toxin from Absorption or digestion by the animals.

Layer of weter molecules adhere to certain compounds of the feed additives attracts Mycotoxins, like Aflatoxin, that have functional polar atomic group. The adsorbed Mycotoxins thus are isolated from the digestive process and later excreted. Most of these products are designated to sequester or trop toxin molecules during digestion of nutrient absorption in order to prevent Pathological effects in the animals.

The different Mycotoxins have extremely diverse molecular structure in this sense, they are similar to vitamins, whereas, all amino acids have similar structure. Thus, it would seem reasonable to suppose that until data contrary is presented any material capable sequestering multiple Mycotoxins is also likely to trap one or more of Mycotoxin or vitamins, minerals, essential amino acids, medications etc. that are present in conventional poultry feeds and are of value for the animals. Data existing which suposedly indicate that products acutally on the market have activity against multiple toxins. However, the interpretation of this data remains an open question.

Use of Enzmes:

However, some of the most dangerous Mycotoxins cannot be inactivated by the use off toxin binders (Additives) as they lack the polar functional atomic groups of the aflatoxin. So to combat Zearalenone and the Trichothecenes, the additive contains enzyme complexes that attract specific functional groups of atoms in the Mycotoxins. The enzyme estrase for example break the lactone ring of Zearalenone while the Enzyme epoxidase degrades 12, 13, epoxy group in the Trichothecene. By breaking apart the functional atomic

Impact of monoxygenase inductors (IMO) in combination with Goba, Metheonine or Zealite on productivity of broliers.

Sl. No.	Added to the ration	Live weight at 7 weeks of age (g)	Feed consumption /1 Kg. weight gain (kg)	Aflatoxin content in of the liver (mg/kg)
1.	-	1968±47	2.10	18.2±1.6
2.	1.9 gm/kg Aflatoxin B-1	1686±31	2.60	10.0±0.9(×)
3.	1.9 mg/kg Aflatoxin +1 MO + Gaba	1827±32(.)	2.45	8.9 ±1.1 (×)
4.	1.9 mg/kg Aflatoxin + 1 MO + Methionine	18510±41	2.23	9.6 ±1.1 (×)
5.	1.9 mg/kg Aflatoxin + 1MO + Zeolite	1897±38	2.24	9.6±1.1 (′)
6.	1.9 mg/kg Aflotoxin + IMO+ Zeolite	1850±40 (.)	2.32	9.2 ±1.4 (×)

(.) Higher compared 2nd group P< 0.01
□ Higher compared 2nd group P< 0.001
(×) Lower compared 2nd group P<0.01

groups within the Mycotoxins molecule the Enzyme renders them non-toxic. As non-toxic metabolites the Edegraded Mycotoxins are digested or excreted without harm to the animals.

Index